ART, SURGERY
and
TRANSPLANTATION

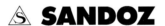

Sponsored by an educational grant from Sandoz Pharma Ltd.,
Basel, Switzerland

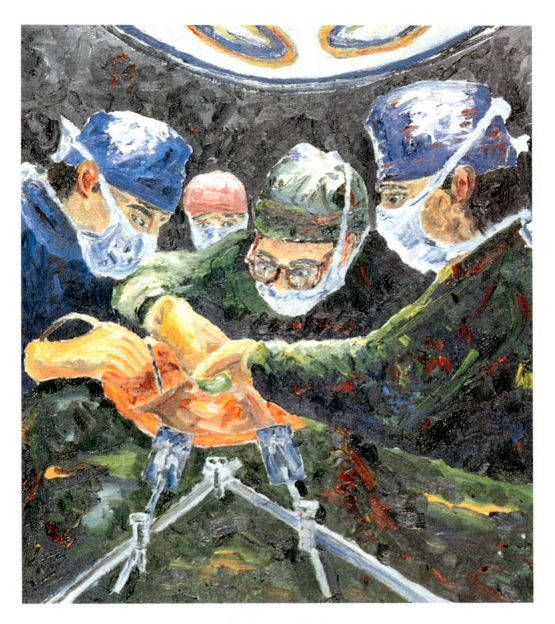

The Moment of Truth

ART, SURGERY
and
TRANSPLANTATION

Sir Roy Calne

Professor of Surgery, University of Cambridge
Addenbrooke's Hospital, Cambridge

Williams & Wilkins Europe Ltd.

LONDON • BALTIMORE • PHILADELPHIA • PARIS • BANGKOK
HONG KONG • MUNICH • SYDNEY • TOKYO • BUENOS AIRES • WROCLAW

Editor: Anne Lenehan
Managing Editor: Jane Smith
Cover and Interior Design: Marie McNestry
Printer and Binder: Artegrafica, Verona, Italy

Williams & Wilkins Europe Ltd.
Broadway House
2–6 Fulham Broadway
London SW6 1AA, UK

Telephone 0171 385 2357
Facsimile 0171 385 2922

Williams & Wilkins
351 West Camden Street
Baltimore
Maryland 21201-2436, USA

Printed in Italy by Artegrafica.

A CIP catalogue record for this book is available from the British Library.

96 97 98
1 2 3 4 5 6 7 8 9 10

ISBN 0-683-23094-8

TABLE *of* CONTENTS

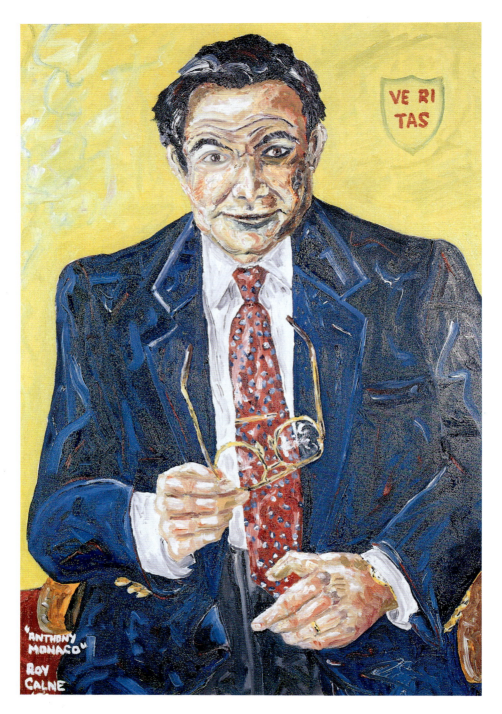

Dr Anthony Monaco, Professor of Surgery, Harvard Medical School and Surgeon to the Deaconess Hospital, Boston. Dr Monaco has been at the forefront of research into mechanisms of graft tolerance in a variety of animals, using a wide range of protocols. He has achieved success in a number of models, which are likely to be relevant to humans.

FOREWORD

MARY LOU *and* **ANTHONY P MONACO**, MD

Our first real introduction to Sir Roy Calne's art took place on our flight from Barcelona to Boston *via* London, when returning from a European Society of Transplantation Congress. We had the good fortune to be sitting in close proximity to Sir Roy on the flight and we had ample opportunity to look at a collection of photographs of his paintings. We were very impressed, not only by his obvious artistic ability, but by the paintings of his patients in which he managed to capture their pain and suffering, along with their optimism; the pictures of the children who had received liver transplants were most touching.

We learned how Sir Roy involved his young patients in the process of creating their portraits by asking them to colour his drawings. It immediately occurred to us that this was a remarkable form of therapy and highlighted the human dimension of transplant surgery; the youngsters were able to view their doctor in quite a different role from the one they perceived as primarily responsible for their pain. Confronting their illness in a visual and less threatening way, can be psychologically beneficial to the patients, both children and adults, and can contribute enormously to their recovery. In fact, we wondered why the large number other surgeons who paint had failed to recognise this obvious therapeutic method.

Most surgeons who paint in their spare time tend to concentrate on pastoral scenes *'en pleine air'*. Such a past-time certainly contributes to the well-being of the surgeon, by acting as a valuable source of relaxation for those who pursue such a demanding and stressful occupation. Several distinguished surgeons have also been acclaimed as artists; for example, Joseph R Wilder, Professor Emeritus of Surgery at Mount Sinai School of Medicine, New York and former Director of Surgery at the Hospital for Joint Diseases, produced numerous paintings in 'The Surgeon at Work Series'. Henry Tonks, who completed his medical training, eventually became Director of the Slade School of Art in London. In addition, the American surgeon, Richard B Stark, produced works depicting his surgical experience in the European theatre during World War II. These artists focused on their experiences as surgeons and contributed to the viewer's understanding of medicine and surgical procedures.

One cannot mention surgery and art without remembering the famous American realist, Thomas Eakins. Eakins studied anatomy at Jefferson Medical College, but later abandoned his medical career. Eakins' most renowned works, 'The Gross Clinic" and 'The Agnew Clinic' deal with the essentially repulsive subject of surgery in a direct way, but also with great reverence for human suffering. Most of his paintings depict more everyday scenes, such as rowing on the Schuylkill River in his native Philadelphia. Such art makes a marvellous contribution to the cultural lives of people and can never be dismissed. Each work of art makes a statement about the period of history in which it was painted and brings aesthetic and emotional pleasure to many people.

Eakins' masterpieces focused on the art of surgery in a stark and realistic way, however, the fear, pain and suffering of the patient cannot be depicted in such an exact representation. It is in this area that Sir Roy extends and enlarges the relationship of art and surgery. Sir Roy's paintings of the recovering patient, full of hope as well as fear and chronic pain, are truly unique. To the best of our knowledge, Sir Roy is the first surgeon to work directly with his patients in creating his art, even though countless artists have depicted the emotional impact of illness on their subjects. Sir Roy's enormous contribution to the science of organ transplantation, over the past forty years, has been further enhanced by this intense relationship between art and surgery. The visual arts communicate a powerful message even greater than the written word; for this reason, we encouraged the creation of this important book.

We had been aware of Sir Roy's artistic avocation for many years, but the first time we actually saw one of his paintings was at the Royal Academy of Art Annual Exhibition in 1988, during a trip to London. The painting was a wonderful portrait of John Bellany, a well-known Scottish artist. At the time of the portrait, Bellany was recovering from a liver transplant and was encouraging Sir Roy's artistic talent by giving him useful hints, especially in the use of colour. The slide show on the flight from Barcelona intrigued us and highlighted the valuable connection between art and surgery. So much so, that when we received an invitation in the fall of 1991 to attend an exhibition of Sir Roy's paintings in New York, we were determined to go. This exhibition, called "The Gift of Life" was sponsored by Sandoz Pharmaceuticals and contained a collection of remarkable paintings of heroic patients which left an indelible impression. We were determined to bring the exhibition to Boston, where Sir Roy had performed his pioneering work using the immunosuppressive drug, Imuran, at the Peter Bent Brigham Hospital in early 1950. The Brigham was also the site of the first kidney transplant between identical twins performed in 1956 by the Nobel Laureate (1990) Dr Joseph Murray and his team, for whom Sir Roy worked. While we were working out the details for bringing the exhibition to Boston, the show travelled to Houston for the annual meeting of the American Society of Transplantation Physicians and Surgeons, and was then installed, for several months, at the National Academy of Sciences in Washington, D.C.

In June 1992, we travelled to Cambridge for two purposes; Sir Roy had invited Dr Monaco to Cambridge as a Visiting Professor and had asked him to sit for his portrait, which had been arranged by his family as a 60th birthday gift. Many distinguished transplant surgeons have had their portraits painted by Sir Roy, among them are: Drs Murray and Francis Moore from Boston, Thomas Starzl from Pittsburgh, Dr Jean Borel from Switzerland, Jean Dausset from Paris, Jan van Rood of The Netherlands, Paul Terasaki from Los Angeles, and Felix Rapaport in New York. We were delighted to be included in such stellar company and were thrilled with the finished portrait, which is now proudly displayed in our house.

Finally, in April 1993, the month of the National Organ Donation Awareness Week in the United States, the "Gift of Life" exhibition came to Boston with the help of Dr Murray, the co-operation of the Peter Bent Brigham Hospital, and the generous financial support of Sandoz. The exhibition was installed in the lobby of the Brigham, an appropriate venue, since the Brigham has contributed to the important advances in the field of transplantation over the past forty years. Thousands of patients, their families and friends, along with the entire Boston community were treated to a fantastic artistic experience, but more importantly, the exhibition increased public awareness of organ donation. The publication of *Art, Surgery and Transplantation* will communicate this important message to many more people, throughout the world, by the combined power of the written word and the visual images.

We cannot conclude this brief overview of our friendship with Sir Roy and our introduction to his art, without adding a few additional comments. First of all, not only has Sir Roy made an outstanding contribution to the field of surgery, especially transplantation research, through his scientific achievements, but his art adds a dimension which should be enthusiastically applauded. Anatomical drawings, photography, and computer imaging make an enormous contribution to the art of surgery. The artistic impression, however, depicting the humanity of transplant patients and those individuals who have devoted their lives to the care of such patients, provides an invaluable method of understanding one of the most remarkable achievements in medicine in the latter half of this century. Sir Roy's talent as an artist is not just limited to the portrayal of surgery, but includes a number of magnificent Chinese style water-colours. We are the proud owners of "Patsy's Roses" which hangs in our dining room and reminds us daily of Lady Calne's beautiful garden in Cambridge. This purely aesthetic aspect of Sir Roy's work is a further tribute to his appreciation for and sensitivity to the miracles and mysteries of nature. And finally, we are honoured to provide this brief foreword for an important book by a dear friend.

Mary Lou and Tony Monaco
Boston, Massachusetts
September 1996

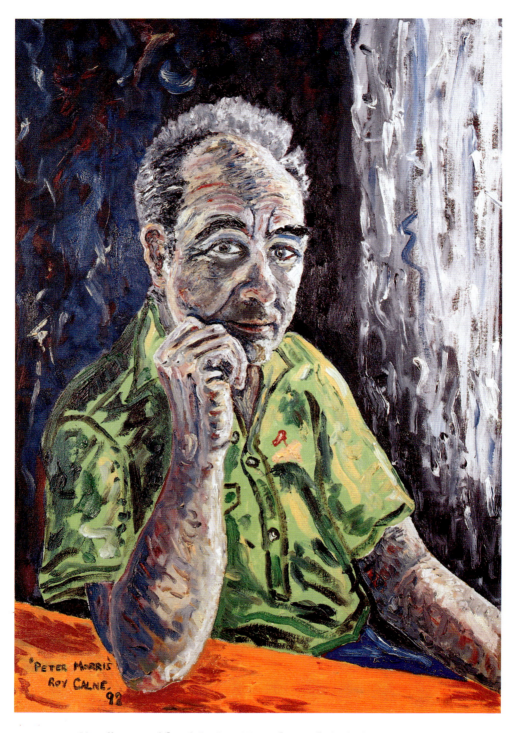

My colleague and friend, Sir Peter Morris, from Oxford, who has established a leading transplant centre in both clinical kidney transplantation and also transplantation immunology. He was a pioneer of tissue-typing and has been a leader in pancreas and islet transplantation.

FOREWORD

PROFESSOR SIR PETER J MORRIS, FRS

This is an unusual book written by an unusual person; Roy Calne is not only a surgeon of enormous distinction and one of the pioneers of transplantation, but also an artist of considerable talent. The subject matter of his portfolio ranges from still life to paintings of patients and surgical operations.

In this book Roy Calne has attempted to depict the association between painting and illness, with particular emphasis on the surgeon's role in the management of disease. The advances in transplantation over the past forty years is a major theme throughout this book, recounted by one of the great pioneers in this exciting field. When Roy Calne commenced his experimental work in transplantation in the 1950s, perhaps not even he would have imagined that transplantation would have reached the level of excellence that we have seen today.

Not many of us are fortunate enough to be able to portray our life's work through painting. Roy Calne's unusual ability to observe and record on canvas, both his patients, and the events of the time in the surgical world, make this a unique contribution. This is indeed a book to be treasured, not only by those working in transplantation, but for everyone interested in the interaction between art and the craft of surgery.

Sir Peter J Morris
Nuffield Professor of Surgery
University of Oxford

DEDICATION

I would like to dedicate this book to my patients who have endured the rigours of transplantation and especially to those who have, in addition, stayed still while their portraits have been sketched and painted. I would also like to dedicate this book to my wife, Patsy, without whose continuing encouragement this book would not have been written.

ACKNOWLEDGEMENTS

I would like to acknowledge with thanks many people who have helped me, particularly John Bellany who started me on the road to painting the story of transplantation. To the Department of Medical Photography, Addenbrooke's Hospital, who prepared the transparencies for all of my paintings. To all those who gave permission for publication of their paintings and photographs and especially to Anne Lenehan from Williams & Wilkins Europe who has worked extremely hard with me to get the text and pictures into a state suitable for publication, and to Marie McNestry for her excellent design of the book. To Cathy Riethoff who has typed and re-typed the text and arranged and re-arranged the pictures. To Sandoz for their support.

Roy Calne
September 1996

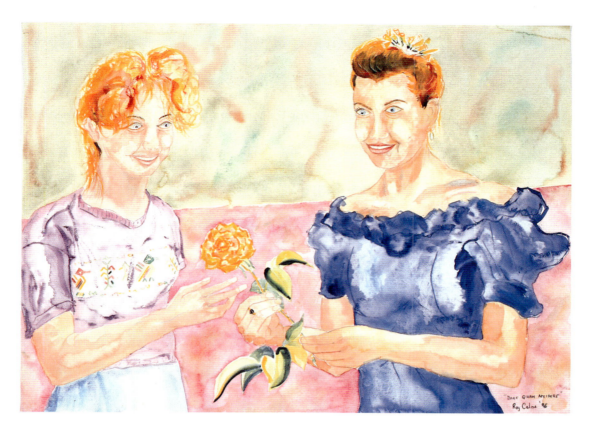

~1~

INTRODUCTION

(1) This picture depicts the inevitable sadness of a cadaveric donor transplant operation. In contrast, I have also tried to capture the joy of the recipient at the successful outcome of the operation. The girl on the right is the daughter of one of our nurses, who was killed in a road traffic accident, and the girl on the left received one of her kidneys. The donor's mother asked for this picture to be a tribute to her daughter and represents the gift of life to the recipient, through the presentation of a symbolic yellow rose. I have called the painting "Dare quam Accipere" (to give rather than receive), which is the motto of Guys Hospital, London, where I completed my medical training.

During my professional life, organ transplantation has been transformed from a dream to an important surgical treatment, even though many aspects of graft acceptance and rejection are still poorly understood. Transplant surgery is now performed by surgeons around the world, and the long-term results are far better than one could have hoped for, considering the wilderness of ignorance that still exists.

The subject of organ transplantation is high on the list of medical topics frequently reported by the media. Very often the operation is portrayed as a technological wonder, eliciting admiration and approval from the general public. In each organ transplantation case, however, there are human factors that even the most sensitive clinicians may fail to appreciate. The grafting of an organ requires a donor, who may be a live volunteer, for example, a parent giving a kidney to a child, or alternatively, the unfortunate victim of a road traffic accident or brain haemorrhage. In such situations, the clinician must be aware of the emotional state of each of the individuals involved – the apprehension of living volunteer donors and the dreadful sadness and despair experienced by the surviving relatives in the case of a fatal accident. There are many hazards during the operation itself, but after surgery there is also the possibility of organ failure due to rejection, infection, or recurrence of the original disease. Even when all factors would appear favourable, a disaster may strike. The surgeon is always disappointed, but also experiences regret at having failed the patient and relatives.

In 1988, the distinguished Scottish painter, John Bellany, received a liver transplant in my department. His first request on leaving the Intensive Care Ward was for his paints, paper and a shaving mirror so he could paint himself in the hospital environment, even though he was not yet strong enough to lift his head from the pillow. During his three weeks in hospital he painted sixty powerful water-colours mainly depicting himself in relation to the staff, his wife and the various events which occurred during this time. In these self portraits he created an image of an heroic figure, rather in the mould of St Sebastian, with the surgeons often appearing as his tormentors, although I believe that this was not his intention.

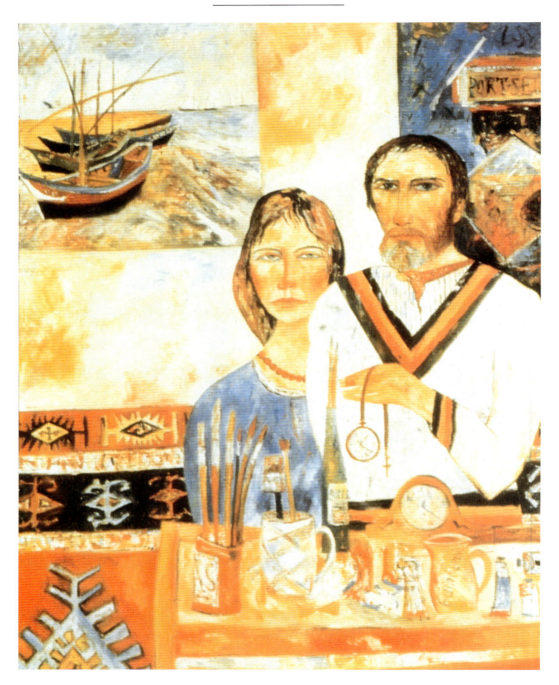

~2~

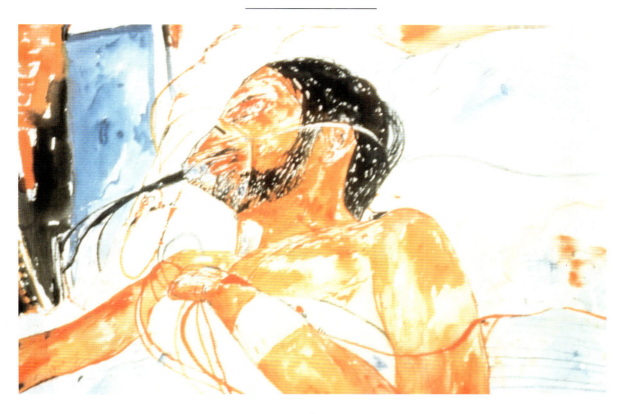

~3~

(2–6) Images of the distinguished Scottish artist, John Bellany. In the first, Bellany and his wife, Helen, are contemplating his rapidly deteriorating condition. The second image is a self portrait, produced the day that he left the Intensive Care Ward. Image 3, which he kindly dedicated to me, depicts the ward round. He lies in bed, recovering slowly, with a stoical expression on his face. In the background are the surgeon and house surgeon discussing his progress. Image 4, depicts the relapse he endured during his recovery period, which required a tube to be re-inserted into his stomach via his nose. Image 5, is a powerful water-colour in which his pain and suffering are clearly portrayed.

I have been interested in drawing and painting since childhood and John Bellany and I quickly became friends. He very kindly gave me some lessons, and passed on a number of helpful hints, particularly regarding his wonderful use of colour. In one of his lessons he asked me to paint his portrait; I perceived him as an extremely ill patient, barely able to sit in a chair and hold a glass of milk, with a long way to go before he was fully recovered. The figure in my painting bore very little resemblance to the heroic St Sebastian depicted in his own self portraits.

I realised that organ transplantation was a subject that had never been painted before since it was a new form of treatment. Therefore, I have tried to portray images of different approaches to transplantation, including the technical aspects of surgical grafting. During the course of painting my patients I have got to know them far better than previously; this is especially true with children, who really seem to enjoy the idea of a portrait session. I am grateful to my models, many of whom were captive, albeit temporarily, in hospital and also to my colleagues and some of the pioneers of transplant surgery, whom I have tried to depict.

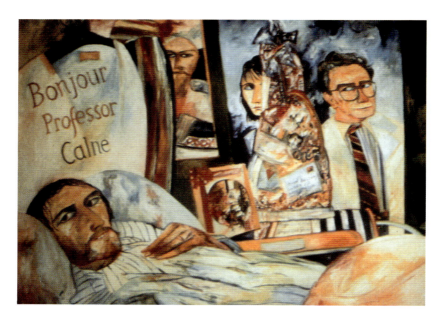

~4~

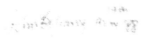

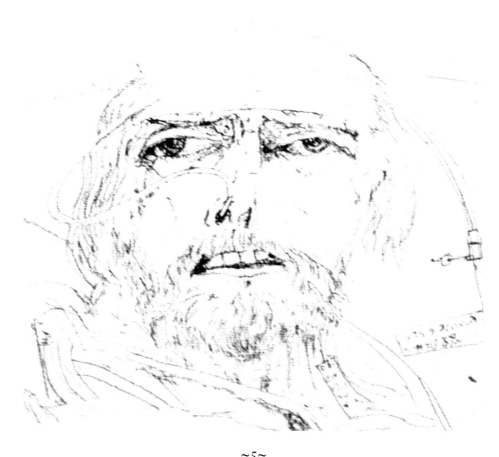

~5~

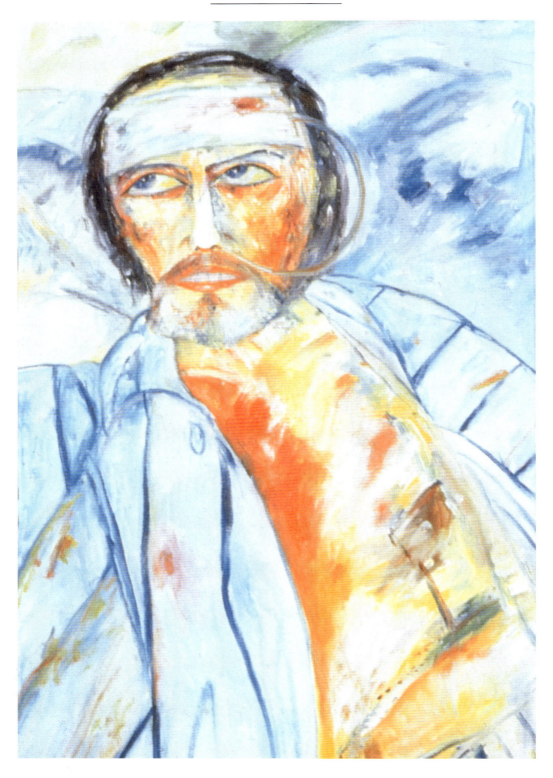

~6~

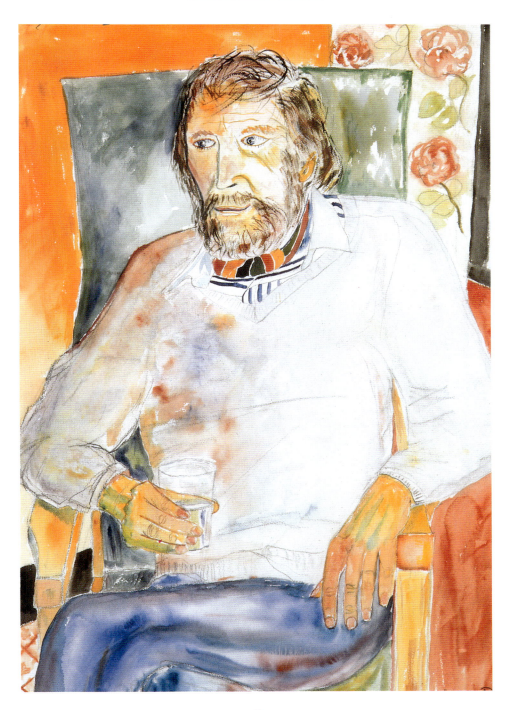

~7~

This is a portrait that I produced of John Bellany whilst he was in hospital.
He was still very ill and barely able to sit in a chair and hold a glass of milk.

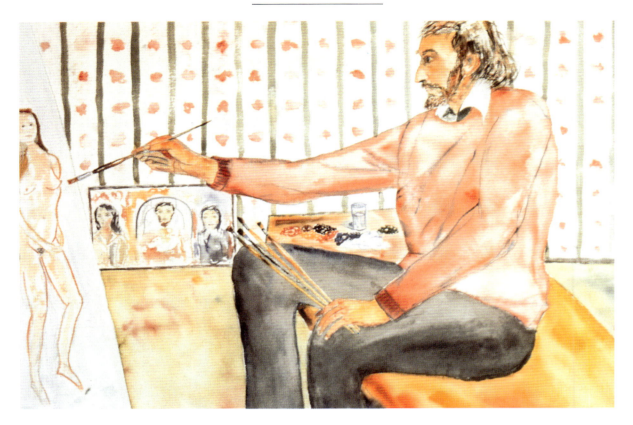

~8~

John Bellany in his cottage near Cambridge. He was recovering slowly, but was strong enough now to sit on a stool and paint. This painting was exhibited at the Royal Academy Summer Exhibition.

(9) My wife and I accompanied John and Helen Bellany to the van Gogh exhibition in Amsterdam and this sketch was produced on the train.

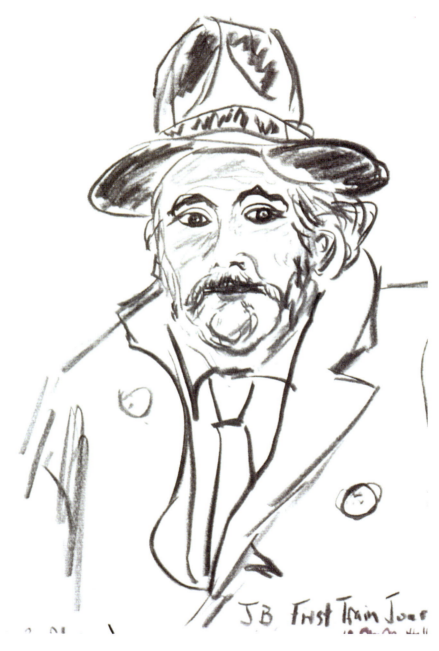

~9~

My old friends and pioneer transplant surgeons, Drs Felix Rapaport and Anthony Monaco, suggested that this subject might form the basis of an illustrated book. In *Art, Surgery and Transplantation*, I have tried to produce such a volume, encompassing not only pictorial images of transplantation, but also the relationship between art and surgery, which has always been close. Both the surgeon and artist need a technical understanding of anatomy, since a knowledge of body structure is essential for their work.

I have also explored the relationship between the doctor and patient and have tried to capture the emotions of those involved, for example, the patient's pain and fear, and their optimism for a cure. I have approached the subject with a consideration of the role of art, especially the visual image, in the context of human nature and nurture.

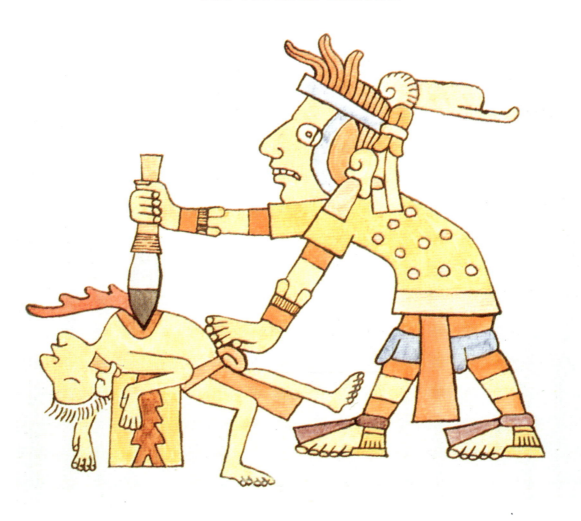

CHAPTER ONE

(10) This is an Aztec illustration of a High Priest removing the heart of a sacrificial victim. This extraordinary surgical procedure was performed regularly and it is alleged that the priests became so skilful that they could remove a beating heart, intact, in a couple of minutes. The modern donor operation for cardiac transplantation takes considerably longer.

ORIGINS

The salient difference between Man and all other animals, including non-human primates, is that we possess the ability to communicate using language. This faculty requires important and complex developments in the brain, particularly the Broca's and Wernicke's areas in the left cortex, and modifications to the larynx so that complicated sounds can be made. The development of speech had important implications in evolution – our ancestors would have had an advantage when hunting and gathering compared with related primate tribes that could not communicate and, therefore, could not plan to work together efficiently.

Modern language has two basic components, namely gesture and articulated speech. There are strong and convincing arguments to support the view that language is an instinctive attribute of the human species. In his book 'The Language Instinct', Steven Pinker elegantly describes language as the single most important reason for our perceived success in developing, what we term, a "civilised way of living together". The distinguished linguistic scholar, Noam Chomsky, has been a leading proponent of the argument that language is an inherited attribute. Children from the age of two or three will learn to speak the language of their parents, or whoever is caring for them, no matter what the language may be. For example, a Japanese infant in a western family will speak the western language fluently and *vice versa*. The child will speak without any formal or informal instruction, but by merely imitating the sounds and gestures of those around him. The infant rapidly realises that the acquisition of these sounds will quickly satisfy specific needs more satisfactorily than screaming and crying.

The next step in the development of communication was the ability to record language in a written form, but exactly how this occurred in different tribes can only be conjectured. However, there are a few rare examples of primitive writing and drawing, particularly where durable materials were used in protected environments. Recently caves have been discovered in Grottes Chauvet in south eastern France with paintings dating back to 30,000 years ago and the most wonderful drawings of animals often in violent action of running and chasing were probably painted 15,000 years ago in the Lascaux region of France. Cave dwellers who lived approximately 30,000 years ago produced the most beautiful illustrations of animals using chalk, earth colours and charcoal on the walls of their caves. The art work is of a high order and clearly the result of training and practice by skilled technicians. The artists were able to do more than just show the main topography of the animals; they could demonstrate the movement and excitement of a beast in flight, presumably chasing its prey or being hunted itself. The purpose of these images, however, is unknown, but there has been much conjecture that it relates to the beliefs and superstitions of these early human tribes. Perhaps they believed that by painting an image of an animal they wished to hunt they would be able to influence the success of their hunting expeditions. Conversely, a violent, dangerous animal depicted on the wall of their cave could act as an omen to keep the dangerous creature away. Whatever their purpose, their execution was magnificent; after 15–30,000 years this ancient art is a testimony that pictures can satisfy an important need in Man. Our forebears must have considered the sight of fresh water or abundant fruit and game as exceedingly happy sensations especially after days of thirst, fasting and laborious travel. To be able to reproduce some of these images for contemplation in their cave dwelling places in winter would give pleasure and this enjoyment would be evident, whether or not the images were linked to mystical, religious or magic rites.

Birds have evolved communication behaviour of an artistic nature that seems to be easily understood by modern Man. The cultural and aesthetic behaviour of birds would seem to be more highly developed and closer to ourselves than can be observed in non-human primates that are closest to Man biologically. The chimpanzee and other apes are unable to produce sounds that can easily be used for the complicated communication of language. The best they seem to be able to do is to scream out and grunt. Bird songs can declare territorial rights, the announcement of a bird's presence, availability for mating or conflict, or give a warning of danger.

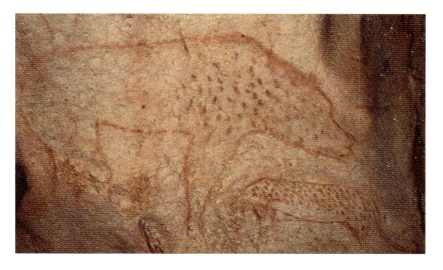

~11~

These beautiful drawings were recently discovered in Grottes Chauvet in south eastern France and are believed to have been produced over 30,000 years ago. Historians believe that the sketches form the basis of written communication. The French authorities have sensibly restricted access whilst the archaeological studies continue.

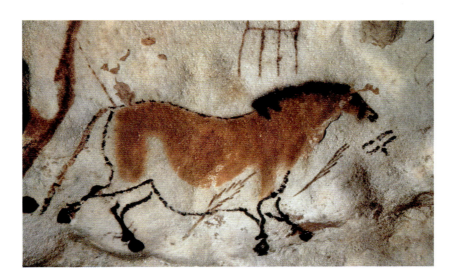

~12~

Early paintings of animals from the Lascaux caves which date back 15,000 years. Like the images from the Grottes Chauvet, these were also produced thousands of years before there was any evidence of written language.

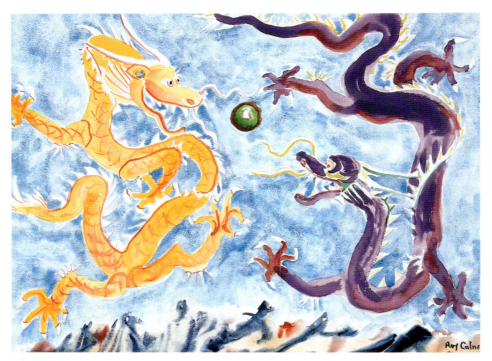

~13~

(13, 14, 15) These three illustrations trace the history of Chinese painting from the picturegram, to the ideogram and finally, the aesthetogram. The first is a stylistic depiction of the two dragons playing with a fiery ball. Initially, only one dragon was to be permitted to enter heaven, but when the deity perceived how unselfish the dragons were, each telling the other 'you should go to heaven', he decided to admit them both. The Chinese dragon, unlike the dragon of the west, is a gentle, playful creature. These stylised picturegrams eventually evolved into the traditional ideogram of a dragon (on the left) and the modern version (on the right). These were drawn by Dr Zhonghua Chen, a Chinese visitor in my Department. Finally, we have an illustration of beautiful Chinese calligraphy, which I call an "aesthetogram". This was produced by Dr Meng-kung Tsai of Taiwan, who very generously presented me with this scroll when I visited his Department. The long tail of the dragon, the mouth and some of the other anatomical features are suggested in the brush strokes. I asked him how long it had taken to produce and he explained that the actual calligraphy had been very swift, but before he started he had to meditate until he could 'think dragon'. I was fascinated by his description of a phenomenon well known to all artists, that good work is unlikely to be forthcoming unless the mood is harmonious.

"DRAGON"

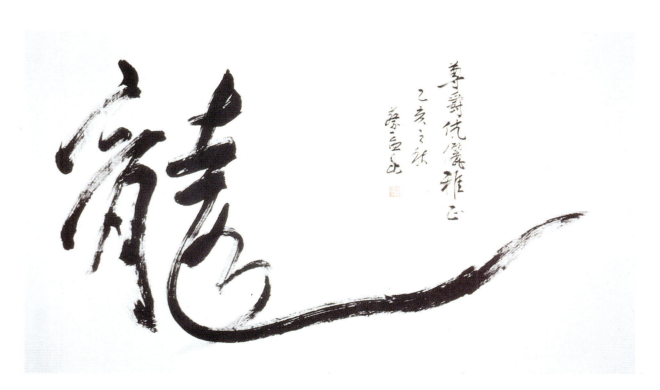

龍

标 standard writing
used by all Chinese

龙

a simplified writing
only used by the mainland Chinese

~14~

~15~

Historians believe that these primitive sketches and paintings represent the advent of communication through writing. Simpler and more functional images, or 'picturegrams', evolved into more stylised ideogram symbols which subsequently developed into a number of written languages. Chinese ideograms were recorded 3,000 years ago engraved in bronze, etched on bones and drawn in charcoal-based paint. The writers of these early texts were not restricted to merely utilitarian considerations; the strokes had a discipline and a beauty that is still appreciated in modern China in the art of calligraphy. From the illustrations included in this chapter, one can trace the evolution of the picturegram through to the 'aesthetogram'. Very often, this beautiful writing is framed and exhibited for its aesthetic as well as its poetic qualities.

For society to operate in a disciplined way, all civilisations sought for, and established, a religious basis for existence. Painting and sculpture played a fundamental role in this culture, for example, the spectacular coloured images and intricate sculptures found in Egyptian tombs. Writing, art, sculpture and architecture played an intrinsic role in enabling early civilisations in Babylon, Egypt, China, India, Greece and Rome to prosper and flourish over so many years.

From archaeological records we have some knowledge of art in these ancient civilisations. Art forms from other early societies, such as the beautiful sculptures of the Etruscans and the early tribes from pre-Columbian America, and the massive stone artwork from Easter Island, are less well documented and appreciated. As well as the religious importance of art and writing, there were obvious secular advantages too in the ability to give instructions for the construction of buildings, ships and machines and to describe human and animal anatomy.

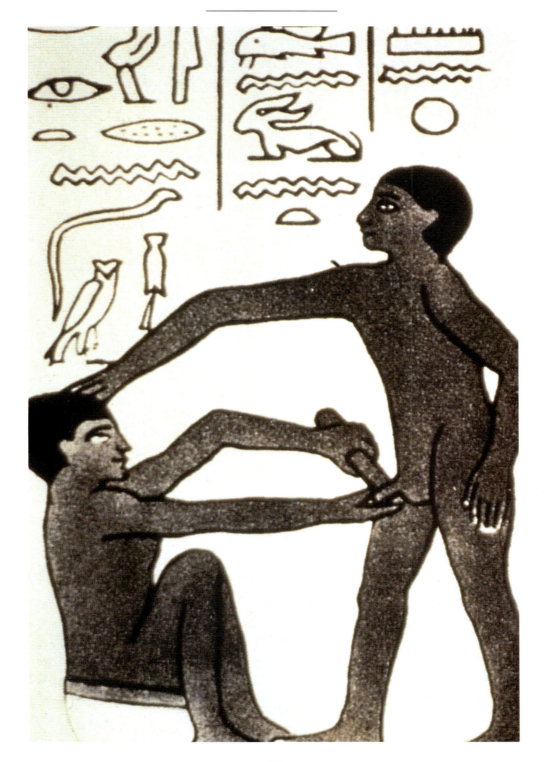

~16~

Circumcision in ancient Egypt. These stylised figures are shown in the traditional Egyptian profile.

The possibility of recording language in a written form was necessary for all the developments of modern science. The phonetic alphabet, together with an easily manipulated system of Arabic numbers, were an enormous advantage in the expression of ideas and the advancement of science and mathematics. The early Arabian mathematicians were able to calculate the movement of the stars and planets with remarkable accuracy, using arithmetic and geometry. The ancient Greeks were the first to develop reasoning, using observation and logical deduction. This, in turn, led to the beginning of modern science, as such skills were applied to new mathematical concepts. The stage was set in the west for a completely new approach to an understanding of natural phenomena. However, the church was an increasingly powerful force and there were many conflicts and struggles to be overcome before natural science could be freely developed. Charles Darwin in his book, 'The Origin of the Species', challenged the biblical concept of creation with his theory of natural selection and evolution, one of the many triumphs that has resulted in the extraordinary growth of scientific knowledge in the past 200 years.

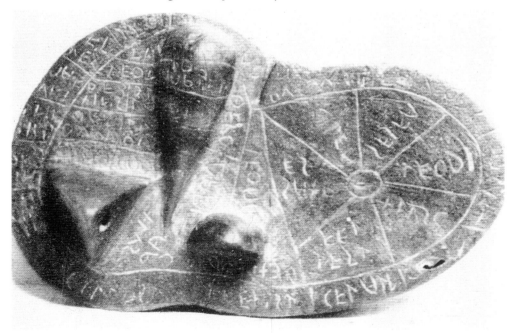

~17~

This is a bronze Etruscan liver. The liver had a central role in the religion of the Etruscans and there was even a High Priest of the liver, called Haruspex.

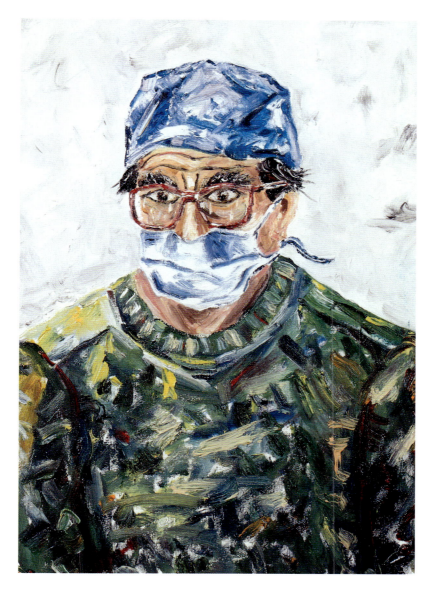

CHAPTER TWO

(18) Self-portrait in operating garb. This was reproduced in the Cambridge Alumni magazine and one of the readers wrote to the Editor, describing the image as frightening.

The URGE *to* PAINT

Like most children, I found great pleasure in drawing and painting at an early age. The subject matter included animals, ships, cars and trains - the things that interest young boys. At school I had the good fortune to be taught by an outstanding art master, Francis Russell Flint, son of William the celebrated English artist, famous for his water-colours of beautiful nudes and partly clothed ladies. Francis Russell Flint taught us to use our imagination whilst painting and sketching and explained that a technical approach alone was not enough to produce 'a work of art'. My love of art also extended to the practical illustration of science projects, especially biology, and I spent many hours drawing dissection specimens and images under a microscope.

As a medical student in London I had an opportunity to copy a Degas pastel in the Tate Gallery. The authorities probably thought I looked shabby enough to be an art student and did not enquire further, but I doubt that a medical student would have been permitted to set up an easel in the Tate. I spent many hours copying the Degas in oils and realised that the artist probably needed only a few minutes with his bold pastel strokes. It seems to me that the blue sash was the focal point of Degas' interest and that the rest of the lines were subordinated and related to this feature.

My interest in painting continued and I met many other surgeons with great artistic interest and talent. A surgical friend in Singapore, Earl Lu, taught me the rudiments of Chinese painting and how to use the Chinese brush. Several of my surgical colleagues in Cambridge are keen painters; we spent some of our weekends with the gifted teacher, Ron Ranson, who emphasised simplicity and a bold approach. His extraordinary enthusiasm was infectious and he seemed to be able to get the best out of his pupils, regardless of their level of skill.

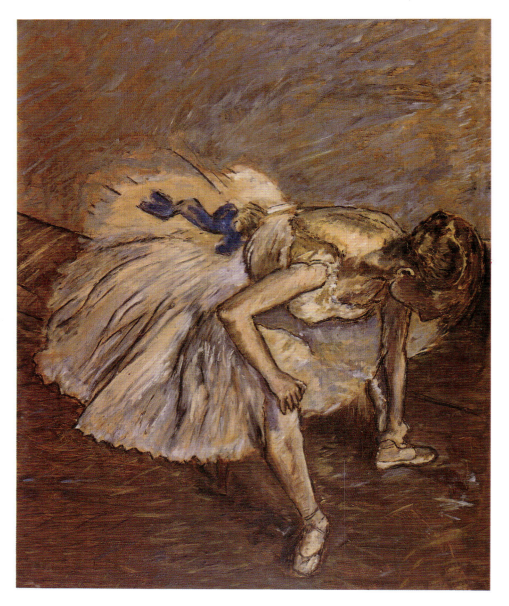

~19~

A copy of a Degas pastel, which I reproduced in oils nearly fifty years ago, when the painting was on loan to the Tate Gallery, London. I spent many hours trying to understand the artist's technique. I believe that the blue sash is the focal point of this picture, and the lines of the ballet dancer and her dress have an important relationship to this feature. I expect that the original pastel took Degas only a few minutes.

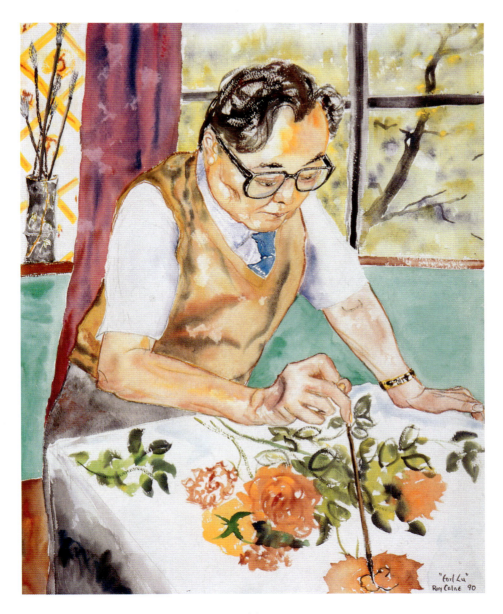

~20~

Dr Earl Lu, a surgeon in Singapore, who taught me the rudiments of Chinese painting. He visited my house in Cambridge, where I painted his portrcit.

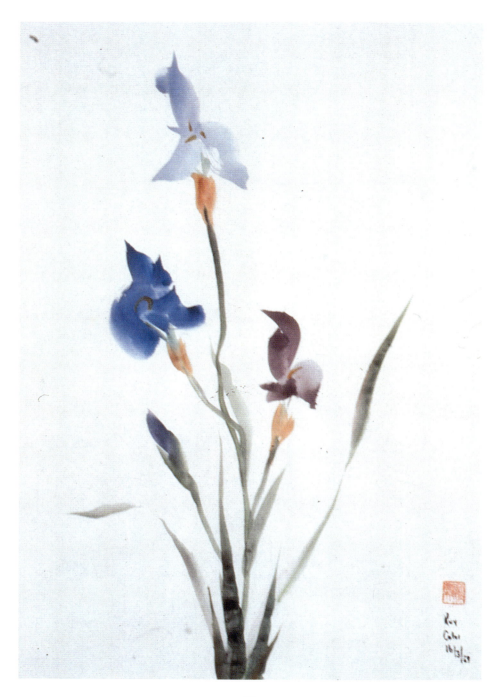

~21~

Chinese style Flag irises in memory of my mother. The word 'four' in Chinese sounds the same as 'death' and this was a tribute to her, hence the four blooms.

I had very little practice or experience in figurative painting until my contact with John Bellany. I tried to learn the techniques of life drawing, but although I have a reasonable knowledge of human anatomy, I found it surprisingly difficult to portray a fore-shortened arm, or the trace of a smile. I like to draw and paint quickly, partly because I am always short of time, but also because models rapidly get tired, lose expression, and move their fingers. I am always amazed how facial expressions can change so rapidly, but always retain characteristics that identify one individual from another.

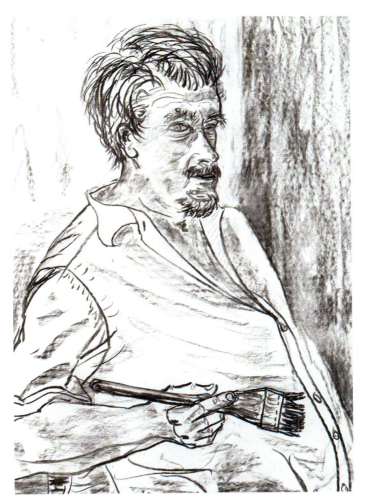

~22~

This is a portrait of Ron Ranson, who taught me how to paint using water-colours. He has a bold approach to colour and paints with a large Japanese brush, called a hake. He liked this portrait, but felt that I had exaggerated his girth!

Painting and drawing have similarities to surgery and research: both require careful planning, skill and technique and familiarity with the available tools and materials. However, a bad image can be discarded without regret; a choice that is not available when dealing with the life of a patient. In both disciplines, the challenge to do better is always present, but perfection will never be achieved.

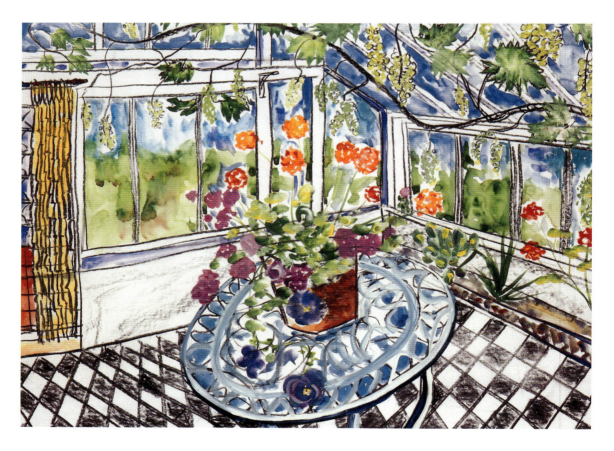

~23~

Ron Ranson's conservatory. This is a beautiful greenhouse with vines growing up to the roof and a chequered tile floor.

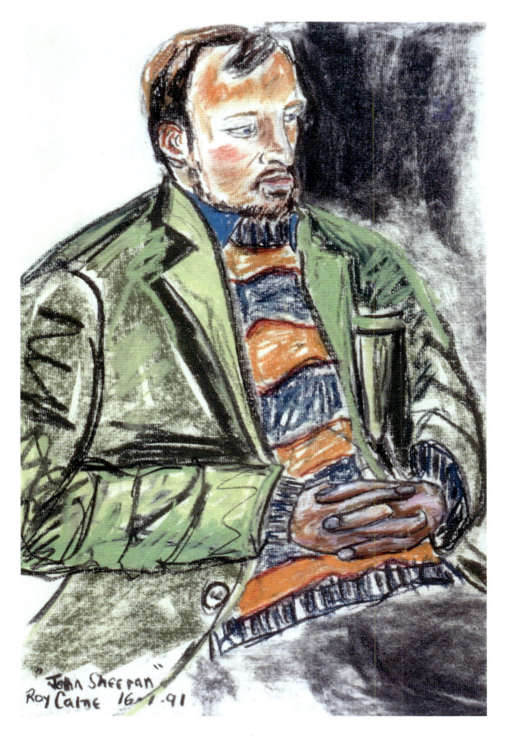

~24~

John Sheeran, curator of art and enthusiastic supporter of my efforts. He has organised a number of my exhibitions and has taught me a great deal about the art world.

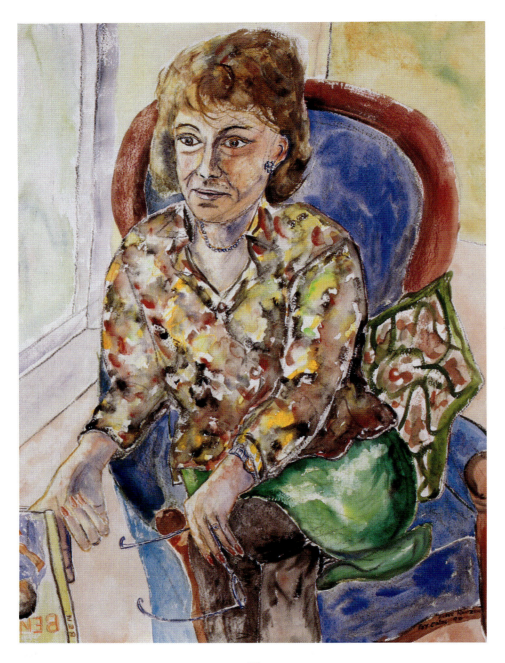

~25~

Esther Rantzen, a well known television personality, who highlighted the case of baby, Ben Hardwick, who needed a liver transplant. At that time, there were no donations suitable for paediatric cases, but as a result of her television programme, watched by some 13 million viewers in the UK, the whole attitude to organ donation changed. We have now performed more than 250 paediatric liver transplants.

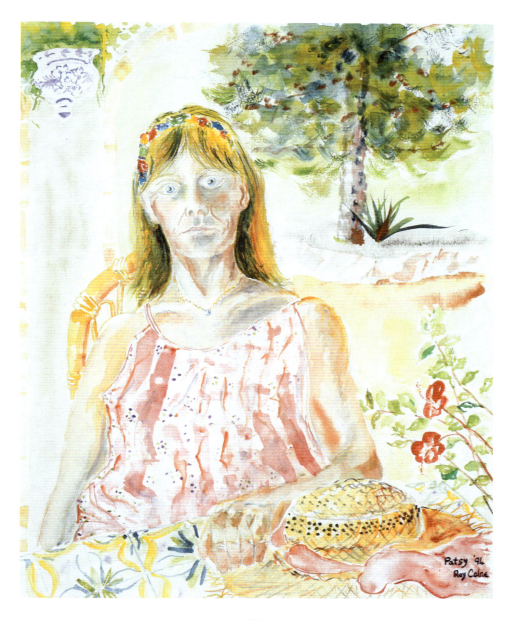

~26~

My wife, relaxing on vacation in Spain.

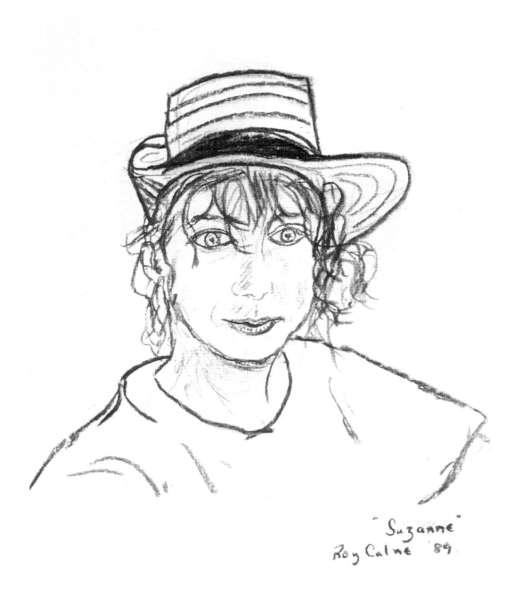

"Suzanne"
Roy Calne '89.

~27~

My daughter, Suzanne, was an Intensive Care nurse and is now an editor of a nursing journal.

(28) Our dog, Daisy, enjoying a run with a bone.

(29) Two master chefs at our College, Mr Sloots presided over the kitchen for 40 years, and Mr Wright for 14 years. It is traditional in Cambridge to celebrate great academics and benefactors, but I think it is unusual for the chefs to be immortalised. I am grateful to them for their hard work, dedication and outstanding results.

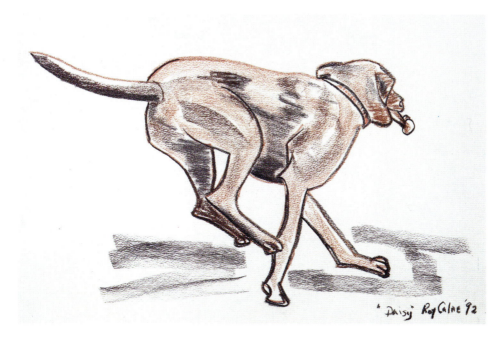

~28~

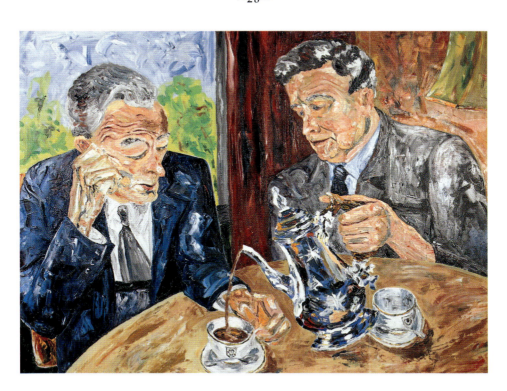

~29~

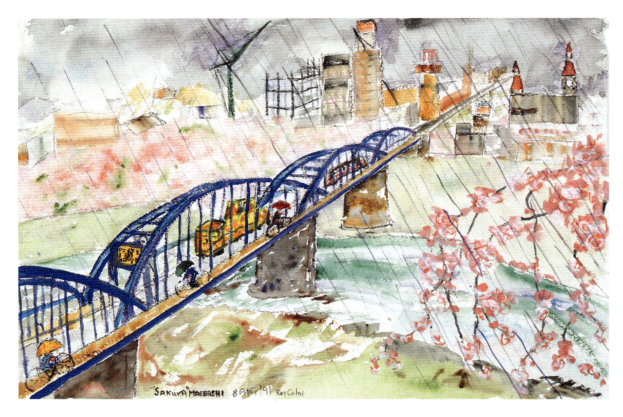

~30~

Cherry blossom, "Sekura", in Japan. This is the traditional subject matter of Japanese artists and was
also used by van Gogh in some of his paintings.

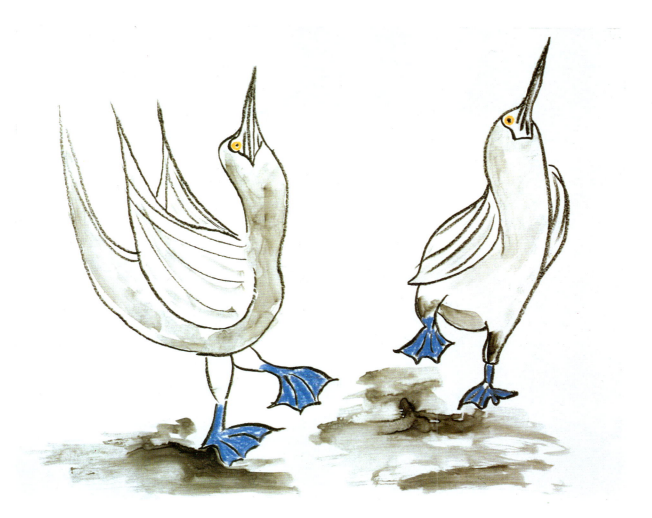

CHAPTER THREE

(31) The dance of the blue-footed Booby Birds. We witnessed this beautiful spectacle in the Galapagos Islands. The female would initially stand still, while the male began dancing around her, gradually building up the tempo. Eventually, the female would join in too, but at a slower pace. We were told that this would cement their relationship for nesting together. If the female was not impressed she remained still and the male had to look elsewhere for a mate.

The APPRECIATION *of an* IMAGE — *an* AESTHETIC INSTINCT?

All aspects of the arts, including poetry, literature, dance, singing and music are "aesthetic", in the sense that they can be appreciated by humans and evoke a variety of emotions, ranging from joy to fear or horror. The word aesthetic means 'things perceptible by the senses', but nowadays the word is frequently used to describe an object as 'artistic' or 'of good taste'. An aesthete, according to the Oxford English dictionary, is 'one who professes a superior appreciation of what is beautiful and endeavours to carry out his ideas in practice'. The original meaning of the word 'art' is 'skill'; however, today's numerous variants of meaning can make an argument about art difficult to sustain without the danger of confusion. Why do we look at pictures? I suppose this question could be answered at many different levels, but the conclusion drawn from almost any enquiry is that a picture triggers our emotions, whether it gives pleasure, excitement, fear or horror. This topic is discussed in depth by Ellen Dissanayake, who marshals powerful evidence in favour of an art instinct in her two books "What is Art For" and "Homo Aestheticus".

Art and, in the wider sense, aesthetics, are found in all communities, from the most primitive to highly developed societies. In developed societies, although attitudes to art vary greatly, the appreciation of quality is something that is regarded as important. Art is practised and enjoyed by all human beings to varying degrees. However, what is regarded as an outstanding creative achievement is, by definition, rare, otherwise it would not be so easily distinguished.

Analysis of the visual image has become more difficult and diffuse. There is a tendency in the west to divide art into that of the populace and "fine art" for the cognoscenti. Fine art has its own "high priests" who interpret and explain what art is to be praised, and why it is laudable even if it gives no pleasure and has no emotional meaning to anyone except, perhaps, the "artist".

However, it may give handsome returns on the bank balance if it is managed adroitly, so that some rich persons can be persuaded to buy works of art as investments. They may have no more interest in the aesthetic aspects of a painting than they would a bank cheque. The dollar sign and the number of noughts at the bottom appropriately signed is for them the importance of the work of art. This is a sad decline from the concept of beauty for beauty's sake.

Since humans can both create and appreciate art, I believe that the urge to produce a work of art must be, in part, related to the effect that this will have on others. It would be difficult, but perhaps not impossible, to sustain a major creative output in complete isolation from other human beings. Van Gogh admired the paintings of others and yet pursued his own original style, but his works were completely ignored by most of his contemporaries. In the whole of his life he was able to sell just one of his paintings. Sadly, van Gogh's brother was the only person who really understood the passion in his works of art.

A sad story concerns a man to whom van Gogh was in debt. He liked van Gogh and, through sympathy for him, he accepted some paintings in lieu of the debt. However, he later threw the paintings out and they were discovered on a rubbish tip. We can only speculate about the effect this had on van Gogh and how much this rejection of his art contributed to his madness. Perhaps if he had been appreciated in his lifetime and sold a number of his paintings, he might not have produced works of such power and expression that were the offspring of a frustrated, disappointed and bitter mind. There may be some merit to the theory that an artist must be challenged to create provocative art work. If we all have an aesthetic instinct, then we probably all have a desire to create images, even if this desire remains latent and is never put into practice.

Evidence of an Art Instinct in Nature

Certain birds have developed cultural attributes that we may interpret as 'aesthetic'. Peacocks and Birds of Paradise have the most extraordinarily elaborate and brightly coloured feather arrangements, which are displayed like a fan to impress and captivate the heart of a female. Another example is the male blue-footed Booby Bird of the Galapagos, who indulges in an extremely complicated and very beautiful dance to impress a potential mate. Having reached the climax of his fandango, the female, if impressed, will join in at a rather more leisurely pace. However, if she thinks that the performance is rather poor she will walk away and the male must find another mate. The red-footed Booby Bird is also found in the Galapagos, but nests in trees, rather than the ground where the blue-footed Booby Bird lives. In this case, the male has a far more restrained type of dance, presumably because of the constraints of standing on a branch!

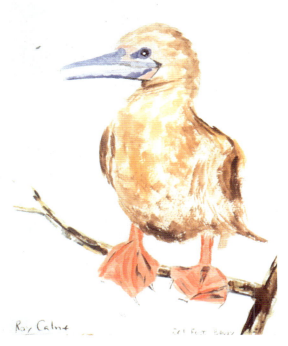

~32~

The red-footed Booby Bird, also lives in the Galapagos, but unlike its blue-footed cousin that nests on the ground, the red-footed Booby Bird lives in the trees and its courting dance is, therefore, much more restrained.

A compelling example of the instinctive nature of art is provided by the Bower Birds of New Guinea and northern Australia. These birds produce ornate edifices of twigs in the form of archways or towers which are decorated with bright flowers, feathers from Birds of Paradise, berries and bright objects discarded by humans. Each species has its own precise method of bower construction. The objects collected by the male are arranged in the bower, whilst the arena in front of the bower is decorated with seashells and leaves. Some Bower Birds will smear the coloured juice of crushed berries or chewed charcoal on the walls of the bower. Having completed a laborious work of art, the male then demonstrates this to a potential mate, whom he will show around the sculpture. If she is impressed with his creativity they will stay together and reproduce. The bower itself has no other purpose; it is not turned into a nest, nor is it used for shelter. It is solely a "work of art", perhaps not for art's sake, but to demonstrate the reproductive vigour of the male. I believe that the creation of art by early Man may have had similar functions, for example, attracting a mate, warning of danger, demonstration of territorial property, and the production of good magic omens.

At the beginning of this chapter it was suggested that an image or sculpture that gave pleasure, or stimulated an emotion, was a reasonable pragmatic definition of a work of art. The academic discussion of the nature of art has been well documented in numerous articles. However, my personal belief is that the appreciation and creation of art is instinctive, and a characteristic present in all human beings, although to varying degrees. The artisitc instinct is a factor in the evolution of a successful tribe, but need not be highly developed for survival. Sensitivity to, and appreciation of, the arts, endows members of a community with an enriched way of life.

An example of the French expression, *trompe l'oeil*, or deception of the eye, by the American artist, Raphaelle Peale, was illustrated on the cover of JAMA[1] (The Journal of the American Medical Association). It is reported that Peale decided to play a joke on his wife, who had a reputation as a chronic scold:

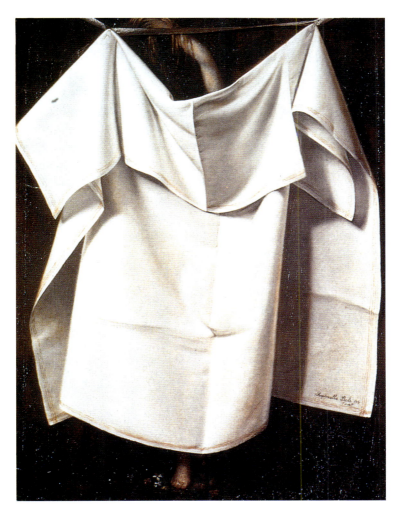

~34~

Venus Rising from the Sea — A Deception. A trompe l'oeil by the American painter, Raphaelle Peale. His wife, wondering what lay beneath her cloth, was surprised to find the cloth was part of the painting, with the girl's hand and foot above and below it.

"Entering his studio one day, so the story goes, she noted that Peale had left a painting of a nude female figure on the easel, or so she thought. The principal area of the painting was covered with one of her best linen napkins pinned to a line stretched across the top of the work. All that was actually visible of the figure was a bare foot in a garden and, at the top, an arm and hand holding some flowing tresses. Furious at whatever sort of indecency her husband had been up to, she approached the easel to rip off the napkin; only then, like Zeuxis, did she feel her fingers not grasp linen, but scratch against the coarse canvas. The work was subsequently lost for 100 years, having been rediscovered only in 1931. Today known as *Venus Rising From the Sea — A Deception* it is at once one of the most witty and most profound works in the entire Peale family repertoire".[1]

In the 17th century, the Flemish school of art perfected representational painting. Rembrandt, the greatest of all north European painters, was able to portray not only a true representation of the physical structure of the individuals he painted, but also the character of the individuals. The importance of the impression of an image in contrast to the exactitude of the representation was introduced by Turner and Goya, setting the stage for the immensely popular school of Impressionism that coincided with the invention of photography. The use of a partial image, or unfinished line, leaving the rest to the viewer's imagination has been used for thousands of years. The Chinese call the line "lost and found"; they realised that some constructive effort by the beholder could enhance the effect of the incomplete image.

The camera obscura was used by painters before the invention of photography to aid the depiction of detailed architecture. There is good evidence that Canaletto and Vermeer made use of this technique, which allowed the artist to make exact measurements and obtain the correct perspective. Photography, with its accurate recording of a scene at an instant, was received by artists with considerable apprehension. Degas put the technique to good use when sketching complicated poses that would otherwise require prolonged and expensive use of models and props. Photographs were used to analyse the features of rapid movements, which could not be separately identified with the naked eye, for example, the leg formation of a galloping horse. However, many artists believed their livelihood to be threatened by the new invention. Refinements in photography have strengthened its utility for depicting the exact likeness in a portrait, but it requires a great deal of talent in a photographer to obtain as much from a photographic plate, as a good artist can do with drawing and paint.

With the advent of photography and other methods of reproduction which allow the mass production of an image or text, the special nature and unique quality of works of art became diluted. This process was greatly accelerated by the invention of films, television, mass produced magazines and the computer. Photographs and videos are often disappointing when teaching a technique. In my experience, the salient points of a surgical procedure may be difficult to define in a photograph, but a sketch or

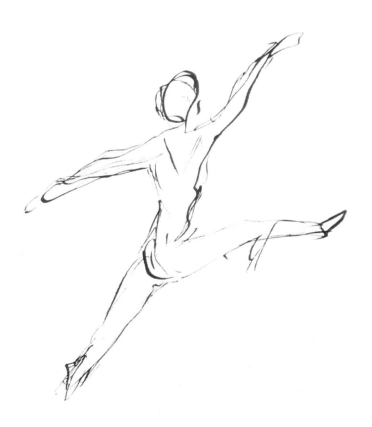

~ 35 ~

A rapid sketch of a ballerina in practice. The lines are incomplete, but they suggest the movement of the dancer.

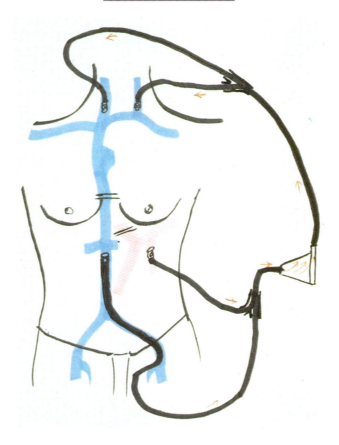

~*36*~

A diagram of a by-pass circuit used in liver transplantation. This is schematic representation showing only the essential features. The circuit takes blood from the lower half of the body to the upper half whilst the old liver is removed and the new organ inserted.

diagram may be easier to understand. A technical artist can sift through the many features of a photographic illustration, leaving only those essential for teaching anatomy or a surgical operation.

Photography is an important component of modern culture and has become an almost continuous stimulus to our brains *via* magazines, television and computers. The visual image is fundamental to the way we live, how we dress, our hairstyle, make-up, the houses we live in and the gardens we cultivate. An individual's image is important in attracting the opposite sex and establishing position and status in society.

Perceptions of beauty change constantly, however, some features, such as the classic lines observed in Greek sculpture, appear to have an enduring quality of beauty and universal appeal. In some African tribes, enormous obesity is regarded as beautiful, whereas in western culture, waif-like models have been the envy of more generously endowed young girls. Despite these variations, a recent computer study of male and female faces from different ethnic origins showed surprising uniformity in the choice of the most beautiful face and it was not the average of many, but certain features deviating from from the mean were considered by the majority to be the most attractive in men and women, by male and female judges, both caucasian and oriental (*Nature 1994 368;239*). These findings support the hypothesis that the appreciation of beauty is partially instinctive and has a strong connection with finding the most desirable, healthy and vigorous mate.

In contemporary society, the purchase of a car is an interesting cultural activity. The quality of the car demonstrates income and hierarchical position. Its design, colour, and performance are closely identified with a self-image of energy, virility and attraction to the opposite sex. No doubt all these criteria were equally important two hundred years ago in the purchase of a horse. There would be a consensus in each community as to which characteristics represented the most magnificent horse, just as there is a consensus nowadays in which is the most desirable car. Why one design is more pleasing than another is more difficult to understand. Just as a painting reproduced too often becomes boring, so the design of a car, if mass produced, can cause cultural fatigue. The purpose of a car for transportation is overlooked in favour of the car's unique style and performance. These are viewed by the owner as an expression of social status and virility.

The Physiology of Vision

Our sight results from light waves falling on the retina of our eyes, like the plate of a camera. Since we have two eyes, each receives slightly different information and what we perceive is a distillation and selective handling of these two images by the hemispheres of the brain. An article recently published in

Nature (1996 382; 626) reveals evidence that the hemispheres of the brain perceive different images; the right-hand side of the brain focuses on the global image, while an individuals' locally directed attention is controlled by the left-hand side. The continuous scanning of our eyes when observing an object or a scene, tends to focus our attention on certain points of interest, and often the major portion of the light rays impinging on the retina are lost entirely to recall. An assailant advancing with a weapon poised will be perceived as a threat requiring instant evasion or retaliation, the whole of the retinal image is concentrated on the approaching threat. This is very easy to demonstrate by asking a person to describe what they have observed when viewing a landscape. Often, one or two striking features have held their attention and the rest of the scene has been ignored.

The subject of perception, and the intellectual and emotional effects of the visual image, have been considered at great length and with extreme lucidity in a number of books by Ernst

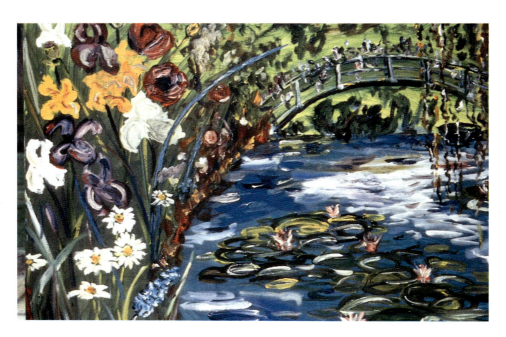

~37~

An oil painting of Monet's garden in Giverny. I visited the garden when the beautiful irises and poppies were in full flower, and this was my impression from a sketch made on location.

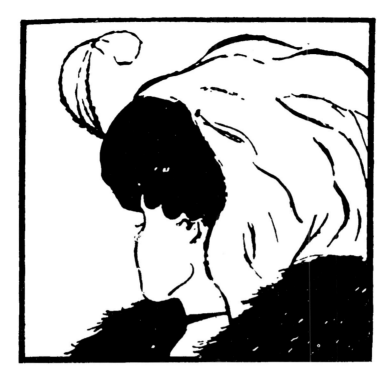

~38~

E. G. Boring's object-ambiguous mother-in-law. She is sometimes seen as an old woman, at other times as a young woman.

Gombrich. For example, if I enter an operating room, I will direct my attention to the anatomy and the progress of the operation. A non-medical visitor is likely to react differently, with a feeling of awe, and sometimes nausea, at the sight of the surgeon's hand violating the integrity of the helpless patient's body. These two perceptions of the same image, by different observers, are individual and subject to marked variation, depending on the familiarity with the scene and an understanding of the action. The 'eye of the beholder' is a well known explanation of this varying response to a visual image. Gregory explores this theme further in his book "The Intelligent Eye", with many examples including ambiguous pictures, one of which is included in this chapter. Many people enjoy these deceptive illustrations; however, I find the switching from one image to another an irritating experience.

The following conclusions are beginning to emerge:

- the creation and appreciation of art are instinctive and were advantageous in evolution as the basis of communication, social cohesion and written language

- the aesthetic aspect of the visual image is difficult to define, even though, most people can easily appreciate the difference between a printed Chinese ideogram and a calligraphic interpretation of the same ideogram. Both would have the same function in conveying a specific meaning, but most people would prefer to look at the so-called aesthetic image.

Art is an integral part of human culture and, without any formal training, humans can identify and appreciate powerful visual images and often relate these to the emotion that the artist has infused into the image, which can vary from the deeply religious to an amusing caricature. Some paintings are easy to appreciate, whilst others require instruction; some reveal technical excellence, yet others are badly executed with a poor use of colour, form and composition. Art may have a functional *raison d'être*, or the image may have been made for purely aesthetic reasons.

In the next chapter I will explore some of the common ground between artists and doctors and attempt to show that the two professions are, of necessity, related and that each can derive advantage from consideration of the other.

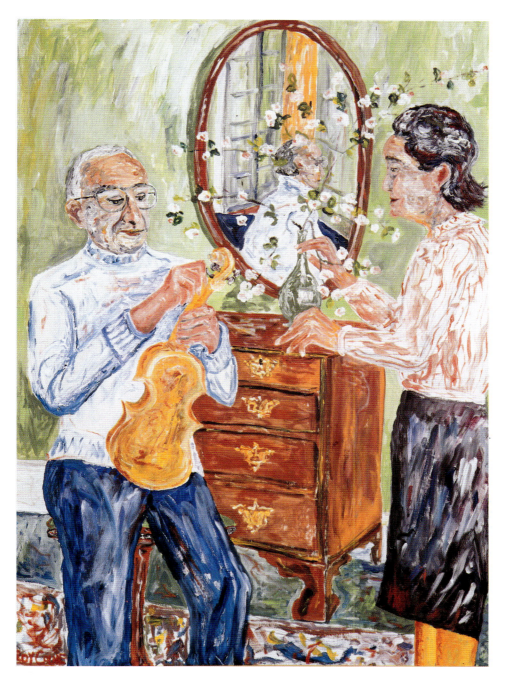

~39~

Ben and Margaret Milstein, neighbours and very old friends of mine. Ben is a thoracic surgeon and taught me as a medical student at Guys Hospital, London.

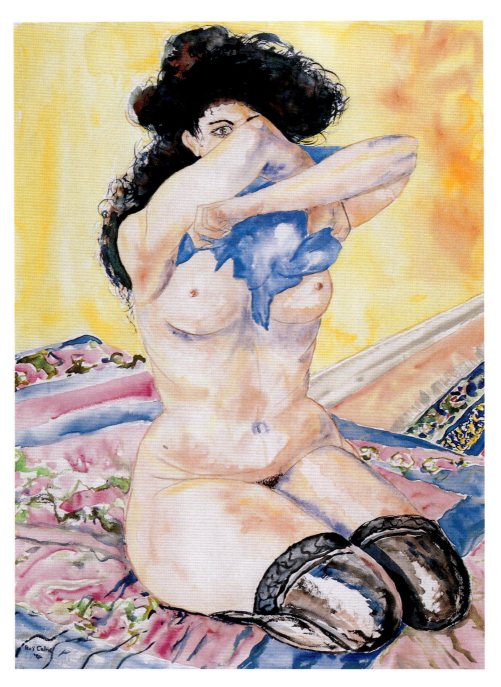

~40~

Semi-nude study with the model looking at the viewer with one eye. The partially clothed body often appears more erotic than a complete nude.

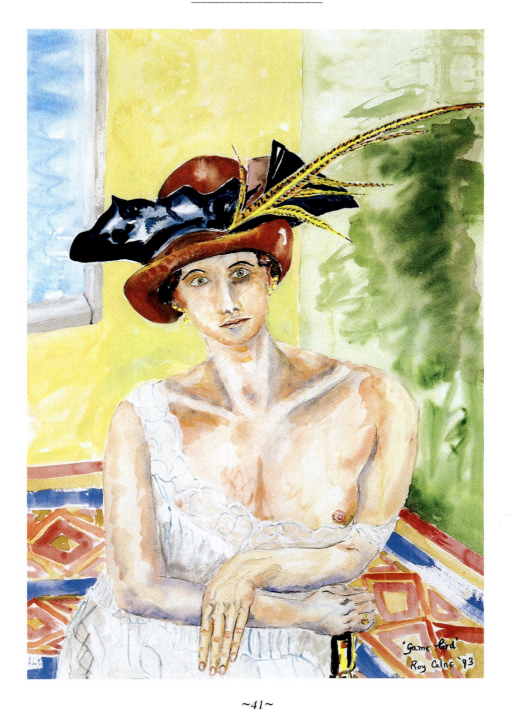

~41~

"The Game Bird". The model, who is a milliner, is wearing one of her hats.

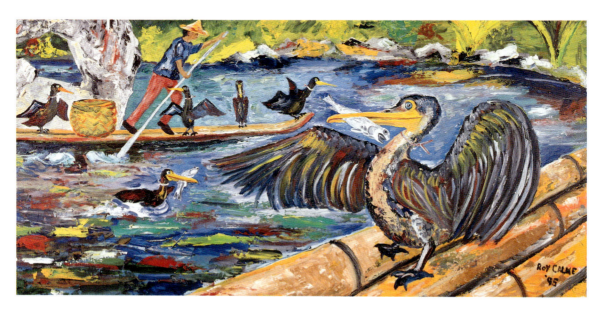

~42~

Cormorants in Guilin, China. I sketched these fishing birds from a little rowing boat. The fishermen rear the birds from the eggs and bring them up as members of their family. There are usually four or five birds on each bamboo punt. When the fisherman gives an instruction, the birds jump into the water and swim at amazing speed, usually returning with a fish in their beaks. The birds have a reed around their necks, allowing them to swallow only small fish. The large fish are taken by the fisherman. This seemed to have some analogy to the way in which certain departmental heads treat their research assistants.

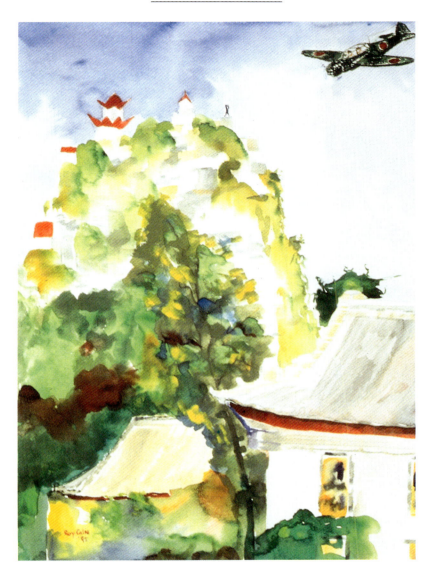

~43~

Some years ago I was invited to be Wilson Wang Professor in Hong Kong and to give a series of lectures. Whilst there, I met the philanthropist, Wilson Wang, who has devoted a great deal of his fortune towards education. He asked if I would paint this tower hill in Guilin as it held special childhood memories for him. As a boy, during the war, he used to climb to the top of the tower to watch the Japanese dive bombers approach. The young Wilson Wang can just be seen on the top of the tower facing the marauding bomber.

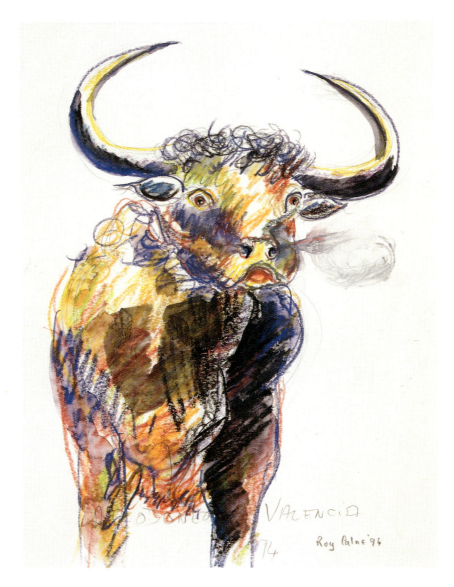

~44~

This is a sketch of a famous bull from Valencia. The bull's head was preserved in a bar and I sketched it there with crayons.

(45) *Threshing grain in Bali. I witnessed this primitive method of threshing grain during my visit to Bali. This oil painting was commissioned for an Indonesian restaurant in Singapore.*

(46) *The Japanese doll. This is an impression, in oils, of a Japanese doll presented to me by a visiting Fellow from Japan.*

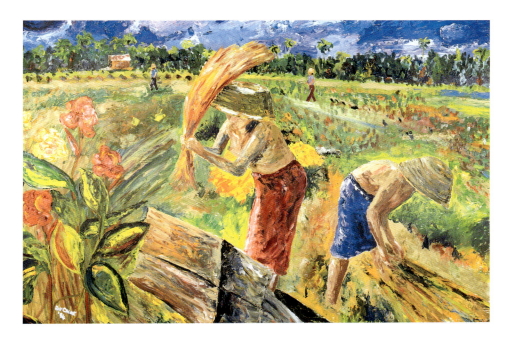

~45~

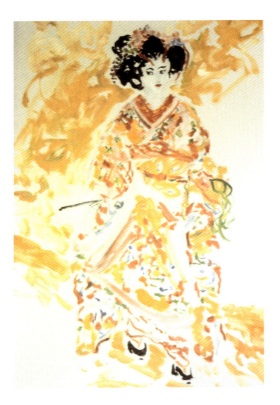

~46~

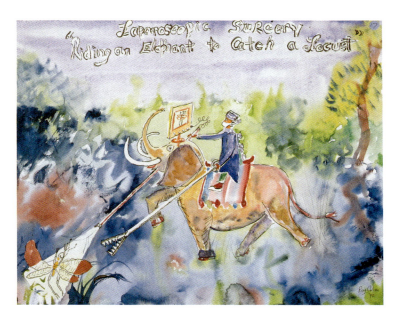

~47~

When I was in Thailand, discussing with surgical colleagues the laparoscopic keyhole method of removing the gall bladder, they told me that there was an old saying in Thailand that doing something easy in a difficult way was like, "hunting a locust on an elephant". In my painting I have depicted the laparoscopic surgeon pursuing the locust indirectly with a television screen, whilst standing on an elephant.

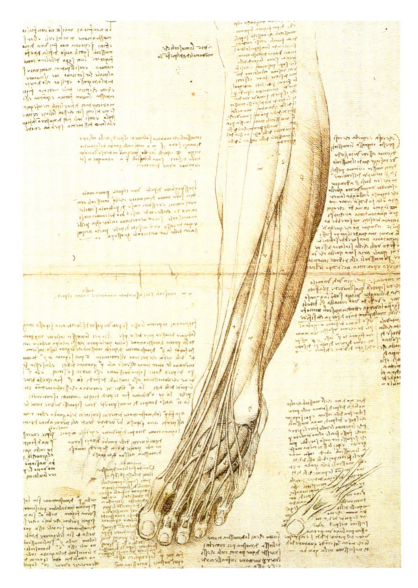

CHAPTER FOUR

(48) A drawing of a dissected leg by Leonardo daVinci. A beautiful illustration of anatomy, which is a valuable record for medical purposes and has obvious aesthetic qualities.

ANATOMY *and* RENAISSANCE ART

Most early art forms were related to religious beliefs and practices and tended to follow a prescribed pattern, lacking perspective, but often with beautiful treatment of colour. The rhythm of drums, singing, the making of music, dancing, reciting poetry, constructing sculptures and totems, painting and drawing are found in all primitive peoples, past and contemporary. The religious ceremonies were often connected with birth, death and fertility of the individuals and also of their animals and crops. A separation of secular from religious culture first occurred in Ancient Greece and then in western civilisation after the Renaissance. It was during the Renaissance that a major change took place, with the introduction of perspective and realism, especially in figurative painting. In addition, a separation of secular from religious culture, which first occurred in Ancient Greece, took place during this era. It was now possible to use the visual image for two distinct, but often related purposes; firstly, to record and communicate information, for example, a map, or the plans for a building, and secondly, art produced purely for its aesthetic value, often referred to as "fine art". The greatest genius of these two facets of art was Leonardo da Vinci, an acclaimed sculptor and painter. He had a supreme knowledge of anatomy, for his time, and his technical anatomical drawings are suffused with a beauty that is apparent even to a casual observer.

A knowledge of anatomy is an essential pre-requisite in order to paint or sculpt the human body convincingly. From observing the outside of the body it is possible to render fine paintings, but a knowledge of bone, muscle and tendon structure beneath the skin gives the artist confidence. Since human and animal forms have figured prominently in art through the ages, it is not surprising that artists would have a common interest with surgeons in learning the basic structure of the body. However, until the dissection of bodies became an accepted subject of study, very little was known about mammalian anatomy and structure.

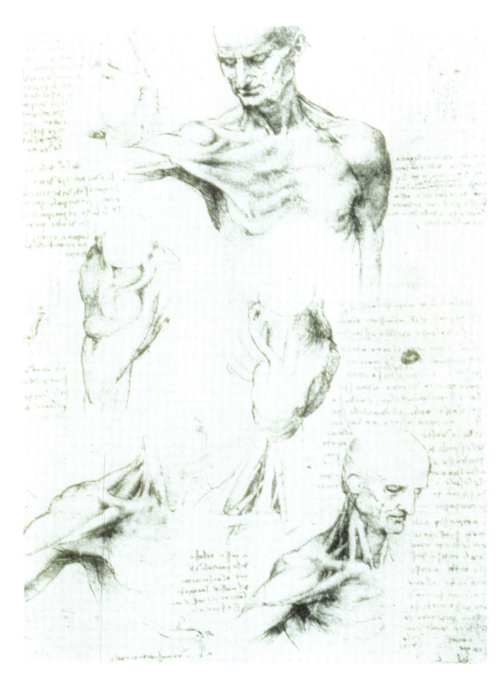

~49~

Drawings of anatomical dissections of the head, neck and shoulder; these images contain similar characteristics to the leg dissection by Leonardo.

The Greek philosopher, Aristotle, amassed an extraordinary volume of literature on the anatomy of many different species. His writings were passed down from generation to generation and, like a Chinese whisper, inaccuracies were repeated and exaggerated. It was only when doctors were permitted to practice human dissection that our knowledge of anatomy increased and people started to question Aristotle's dogma. The beautiful anatomical prints of Vesalius were disseminated throughout Europe after a perilous journey of the original wood blocks over the Alps to Basel. Many of the most famous artists, such as Raphael, Michelangelo, Titian, Rembrandt and Caravaggio used this knowledge of human anatomy to great effect in their works of art.

The Renaissance was also a period of scientific development; doctors and scientists studied the relationship between the structure and function of certain organs, particularly to obtain an idea of how trauma and disease could interfere with both the anatomy and physiology of a patient. One of the most important physiological discoveries at this time was the true nature of blood circulation and the functioning of the chambers of the heart, the valves and the one way flow in the veins. Harvey, a medical graduate of Cambridge, went to study in Padua, a centre of excellence in anatomy and physiology. He returned to England and produced his seminal work on the circulation of the blood in which he refuted the early theories regarding the ebb and flow of blood around the body. Harvey proved that blood must move from the arteries to the veins *via* minute vessels, called capillaries, although at the time these could not be seen. There was little initial benefit to the patient from these revelations, but gradually, an understanding of structure and biological function developed, enabling therapeutic advances to occur.

The coming together of art and medicine in the Renaissance was a necessary step towards the liberation of both subjects, from the previous conventions and restrictions imposed by the church and society. During this period, many outstanding works of art were commissioned and were displayed in numerous public buildings. Scientific observation and experiment yielded tremendous results, one being the understanding of anatomy and physiology. It was only with this essential knowledge that reliable and effective treatments for disease and injury could be developed.

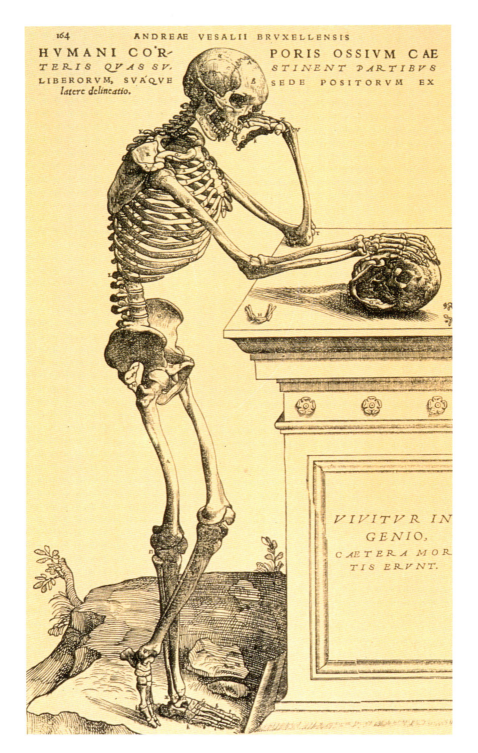

~50~

Allegorical figure by Vesalius.

The medical advances of the 20th century have overshadowed all previous attempts to treat illness and disability; for example, the introduction of aseptic surgery, anaesthesia, antibiotics and the substitution of organ functions by machines, in particular the heart-lung bypass for cardiac surgery, the artificial kidney, and the grafting of vital organs.

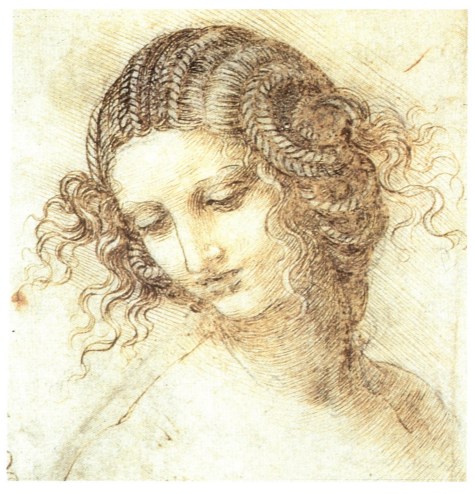

~51~

A beautiful, sensitive drawing of a girl's head by Leonardo.

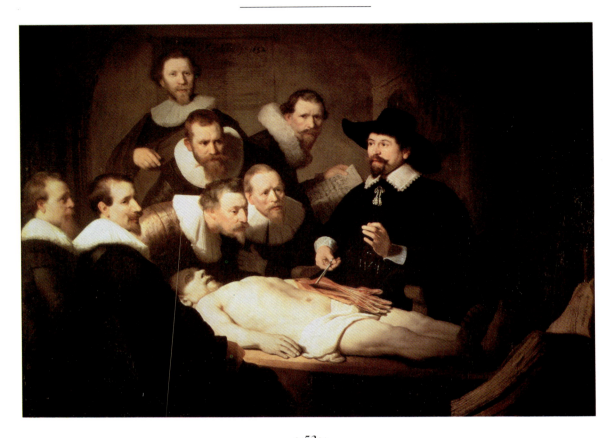

~52~

Anatomical dissection by Professor Tulp. This painting was produced by Rembrandt, who was a friend of the surgeon.

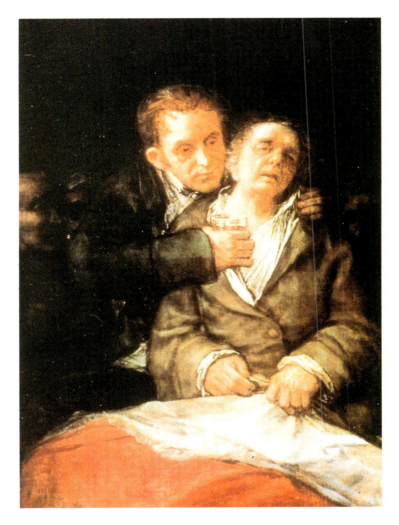

~53~

CHAPTER FIVE

(53) The artist, Goya, developed a serious illness when he was in his 60's. When he recovered he painted this portrait as a tribute to his doctor; he has also written his thanks on the canvas.

IMAGES *of* SICKNESS, ANATOMY *and* SURGERY

Many artists have painted the sick. Gabriel Metsu, for example, painted a mother and sick child. Picasso sketched the inmates of a local hospital and executed a studio oil painting called 'Charity', in which the dying child is probably a tribute to his sister. Edward Munch was deeply wounded emotionally by the death of his sister and he painted this scene several times.

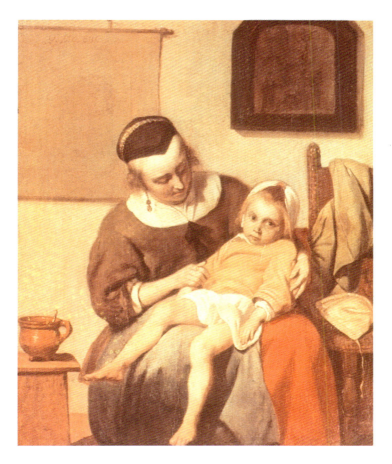

~54~

"The Sick Child" by Gabriel Metsu, which is exhibited in the Rijksmuseum in Amsterdam.

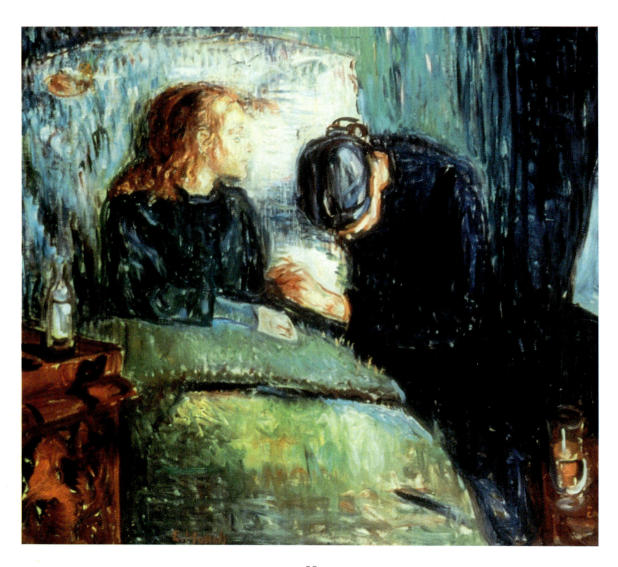

~55~

A beautiful painting by Munch which is displayed in the Tate Gallery. The juxtaposition of warm green and red is particularly effective here.

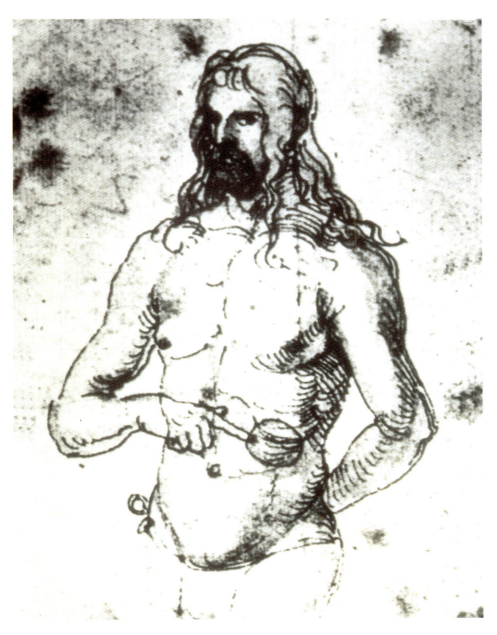

~56~

Sketch by Dürer which he sent to his doctor and asked him for medicine to cure his complaint. It is not clear whether there was lateral inversion of this image, due to drawing using a mirror, or whether it was the right way round, which might help in the diagnosis between appendicitis and diverticulitis.

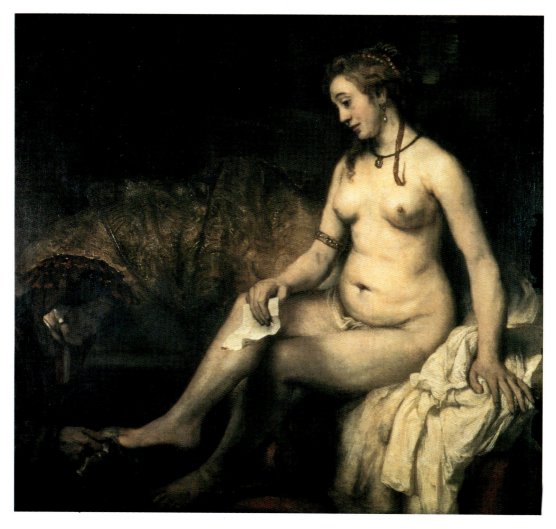

~57~

'Bethshébée au bain' by Rembrandt, which is exhibited in the Louvre. The painting shows the dimpling of the left breast, which probably indicates an underlying carcinoma.

(58) A beautiful drawing of a hand, by William Skelton, indicating cowpox lesions.

(59) My friend, Harold Crock, an Australian orthopaedic surgeon, has spent more than forty years producing a beautifully illustrated book on the vascular anatomy of the skeleton and spinal cord. This is a photograph of an injection specimen of the spinal cord, with the injected veins appearing white.

(60) Photograph of the viscera in the upper right abdomen. It may not be easy to determine all the anatomical features from this picture, but it has a special beauty to me, as a surgeon.

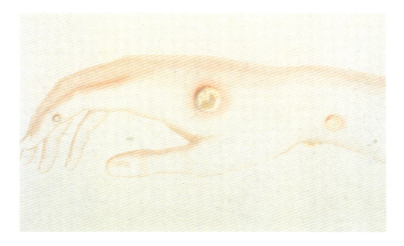

~58~

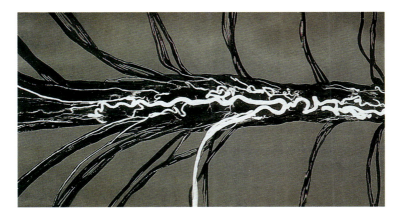

~59~

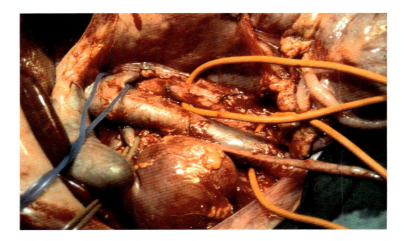

~60~

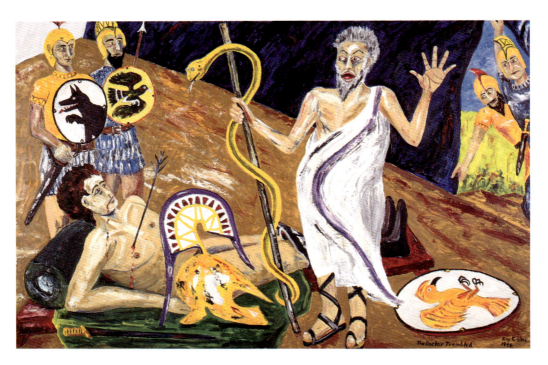

~61~

The doctor trembles. This is my impression of the physician, Critodemus, suddenly being confronted by Alexander the Great's apparently mortal wound. Alexander had led his troops from the front and when storming Multan, a fortified city in India, Alexander and two companions scaled a ladder to reach the rampart of the city wall. The heroic Alexander fought with expected bravery, but eventually an enemy archer shot an arrow into Alexander's chest at point blank range. The ancient texts are of medical interest, since this is probably the first description of a traumatic pneumathorax to be recorded:

"Alexander was struck right through the corselet into his breast over the lung, so that, according to Ptolemy, breath together with blood shot forth from the wound."[2] "Alexander was carried to his tent. Critodemus, a physician of Cos by birth of the family of Aesculapius, was terrified in the face of such great risk, dreaded to put his hand to the work, lest the result of the treatment, if unsuccessful, might recoil upon his own head. The king observed that he was weeping and near to fainting from fear and anxiety and said: 'For what and for how long are you waiting, and why do you not free me as soon as possible from this pain and let me at least die? Do you perhaps fear that you may be blamed because I have received an incurable wound?' But Critodemus, having at last ended his fear, or concealed it, began to urge that he let himself be held while he was withdrawing the point; that even a slight movement of his body would be dangerous. When the king had assured him that there was no need of any to hold him, he kept his body motionless, as had been ordered"[3]. Presumably his numerous previous injuries or chest infections had resulted in pleuradesis so that the lung was not able to collapse.

In addition, the trembling doctor reminds me of an early liver transplant operation that I performed. The patient was lying in the anaesthetic room waiting for her operation and I held her hand to give her reassurance. She looked up at me and said 'don't be so worried Professor, I will be all right'.

Goya is one of the artists I most admire for his dramatic portrayal of human courage and emotion. His paintings during the war encapsulated the brutality of battle and the dreadful cruelty inflicted by man on his fellow men. He was an artist of transparent honesty which is one of the reasons why the Inquisition decided to investigate him. He suffered from bouts of melancholy throughout his life, but in his 60's he became ill with a

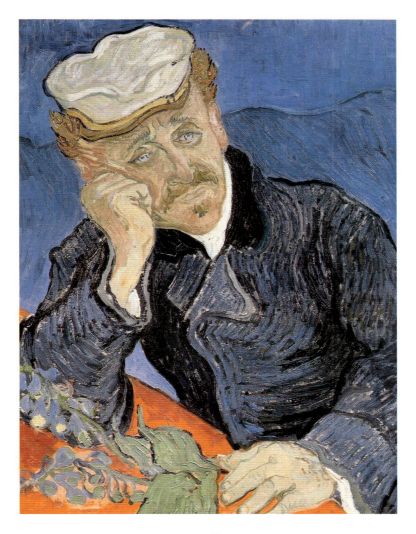

~62~
Dr Gachet, painted by his friend, van Gogh.

[2]Arrian. Anabasis of Alexander, VI. 9. 5-10 2, p131
[3]Quintus Curtius. History of Alexander IX v.24-30 p 413

physical illness that could not be diagnosed. Goya painted a generous epitaph for the doctor who looked after him.

Van Gogh was also haunted by mental disease and fits of melancholy. In one such period of depression, he cut off his ear and sent it to his girlfriend. He became close friends with his physician, Dr Gachet, and lived with him in the final years of his life. Dr Gachet taught van Gogh the art of engraving and encouraged

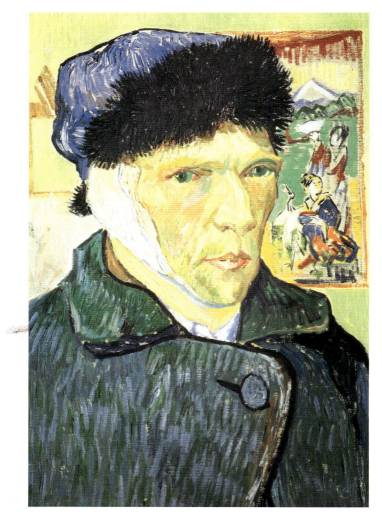

~*63*~

A self portrait by van Gogh, after he had successfully amputated his own ear.

his friend's artistic expression. When the artist shot himself, Dr Gachet looked after him until he died and then, as a memorial, he drew a portrait of van Gogh in a simple charcoal outline.

Both van Gogh and Gauguin were despised or ignored by the art establishment and were difficult characters in their social relations. The two artists perceived a common hostile art establishment and they became friends. Van Gogh invited Gauguin to paint with him and subsequently Gauguin came to Arles where van Gogh produced the wonderful paintings of his stark bedroom and the billiard hall. Gauguin also painted the billiard hall and van Gogh painted Gauguin at work. A story is told of a misunderstanding between the two, during which van Gogh hurled himself at the bewildered and startled Gauguin with a knife. This was the end of their friendship and Gauguin departed the city rapidly.

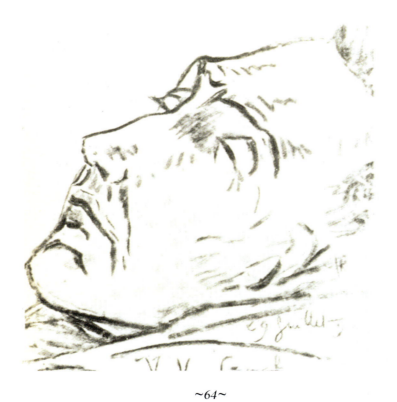

~64~

A charcoal sketch of van Gogh, by his physician, Dr Gachet, following the artist's death at Dr Gachet's house.

Many surgeons paint; I suspect that this is because there are technical similarities in surgery and painting and that drawings are a useful way to communicate the details of a surgical procedure. In addition, many well recognised artists have completed medical training and this affects their choice of subject.

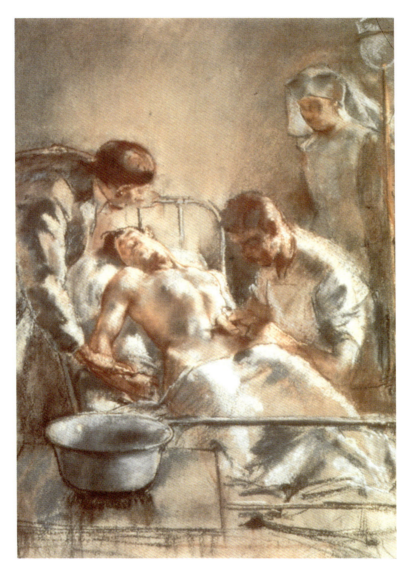

~65~

Henry Tonks. A casualty clearing station during World War I. Tonks was a war surgeon, who worked with the plastic surgeon, Harold Gillies. He later became a professional artist and Professor of Art at the Slade in London.

Henry Tonks, who later became Professor of Art at the Slade in London, initially trained as a surgeon and worked with the plastic surgeon, Harold Gillies. Tonks was a war surgeon and developed his artistic talent by drawing some of the unusual cases with which he was presented. His surgical illustrations are particularly powerful and I believe they may have been an inspiration for Francis Bacon's paintings. The surgeon Charles Bell, Professor of Anatomy at Edinburgh, was also a skilful artist. His famous anatomical textbook contains beautiful technical drawings, which had an aesthetic quality similar to the anatomical illustrations of Leonardo da Vinci.

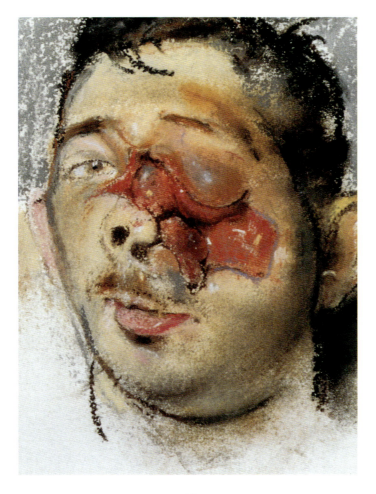

~66~

This image depicts a face prior to plastic surgery. It is one of a series of surgical paintings by Tonks.

Bell was interested in the expression of emotions by facial gesture and published a book on the muscles of facial expression with some fine examples. In one of his best paintings he depicted a soldier dying of tetanus; the soldier had returned to England from the Crimean War and developed tetanus, which at that time could not be treated. Bell skilfully portrayed the dreadful pain of the violent muscle contractions that led to the soldier's death.

(67, 68) Drawings by Charles Bell, which are anatomically accurate and capture the spirit of Leonardo da Vinci.

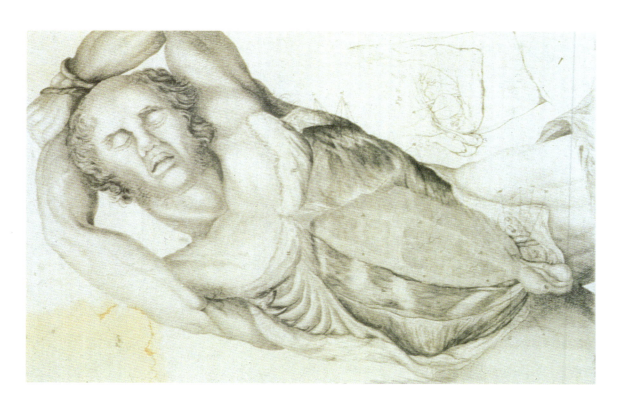

~67~

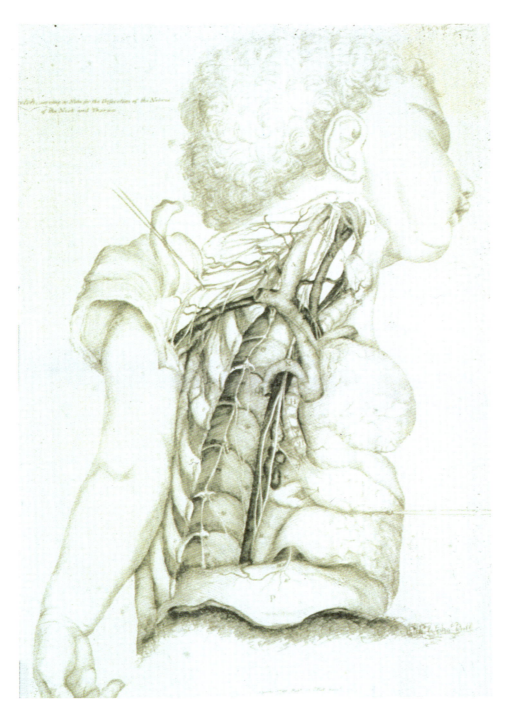

~68~

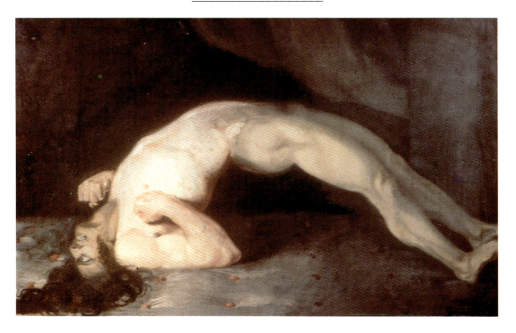

~69~

*A painting by Bell depicting a young soldier, returning from the Crimean War, who had contracted
tetanus. This grim and powerful painting hangs in the Royal College of Surgeons in Edinburgh.*

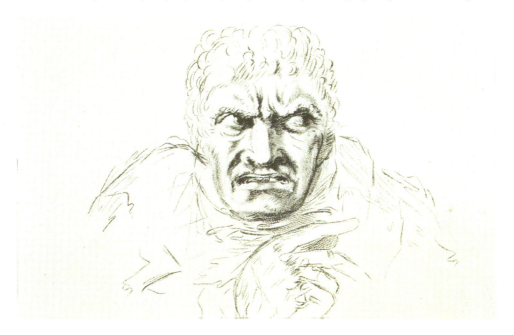

~70~

*Bell was interested in the muscles of facial expression and wrote a book on the subject. This is one of
the illustrations from the book, called 'Suspicion'.*

The Mexican artist, Frida Kahlo, was a medical student when she was grievously injured in an accident. Her spine and pelvis were perforated by a metal handrail when the bus she was travelling in was struck by a tram. The rod came out of her vagina, she was later to explain that was how she lost her virginity. From the injuries sustained, she was expected to die, but she slowly recovered. Sadly, she had to abandon her medical studies, but she took up painting and married the great muralist Diego Rivera.

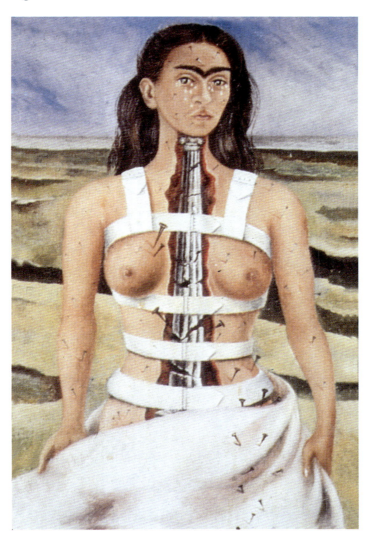

~71~

"The broken column". The beautiful girl is Frida Kahlo, crying with pain from the fractured spine, which she sustained after her accident as a teenager.

During the next thirty years she suffered pain almost continuously and underwent more than twenty operations on her back. Diego always encouraged her painting, usually depicting herself, her suffering, hopes, joys and misery. It is understood that

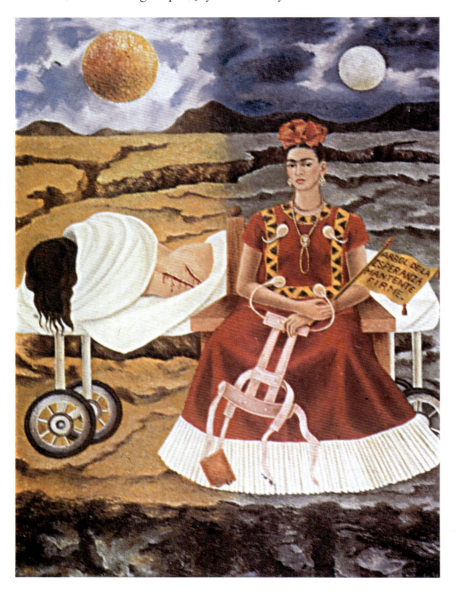

~72~

"The Tree of Hope" represents Frida Kahlo's hope for a successful bone graft operation. The scar over the iliac crest and the second scar over the spine are shown. Unfortunately, she never fully recovered and later developed osteomyelitis of the spine.

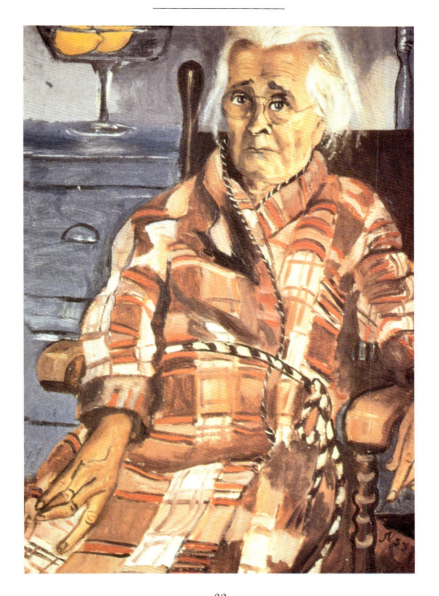

~*80*~

Alice Neal's touching portrait of her dying mother.

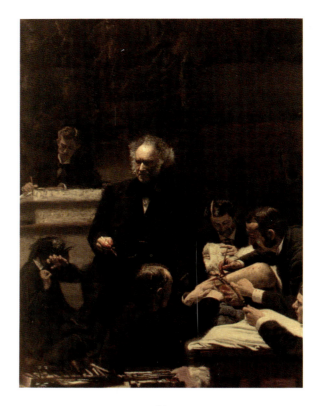

~*81*~

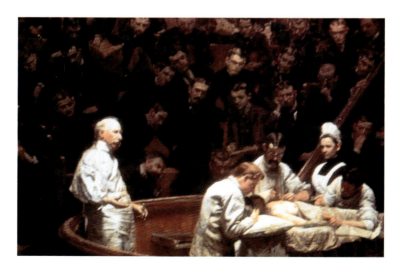

~*82*~

(81, 82) Famous paintings by Thomas Eakins, entitled "The Gross Clinic 1875" and "The Agnew Clinic 1889".

IMAGES *of* TRANSPLANTATION

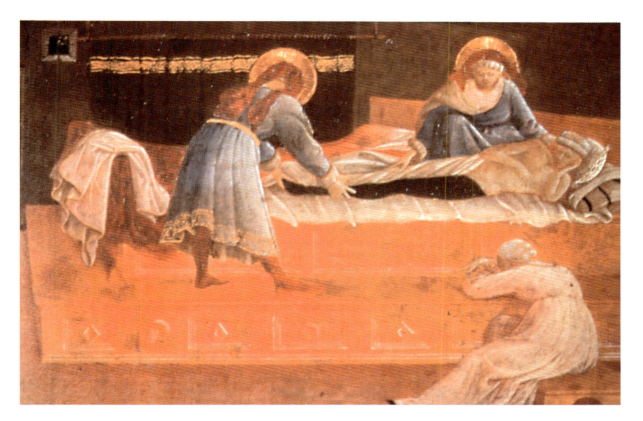

~83~

CHAPTER SIX

(83, 84) Two beautiful paintings by Fra Angelica portraying the miracle of the identical twins, Saints Cosmos and Damian, transplanting a leg to a man who had cancer.

ICONOGRAPHY *of* TRANSPLANTATION – SAINTS COSMOS *and* DAMIAN

Although many doctors and surgeons draw and paint, the subject matter, through deliberate choice, is usually removed from their work. My interest, however, has been influenced by witnessing the extreme bravery, suffering, elation and happiness during the early days of organ transplantation. The idea of organ transplantation stems from the miracle of the identical twins, Saints Cosmos and Damian, who are the patron saints of surgery. It is reported that they transplanted a leg from a recently deceased corpse to an early member of the church, who suffered from cancer. This surgical *tour de force* has been portrayed in churches all over Europe; perhaps the most beautiful are by Fra Angelica due to their simplicity and quiet elegance.

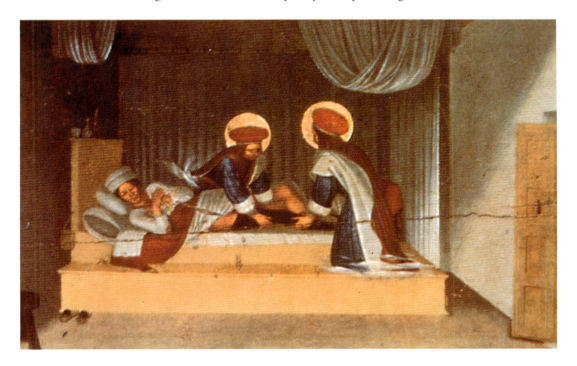

~84~

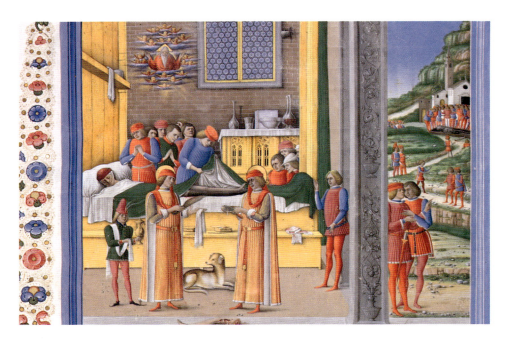

~85~

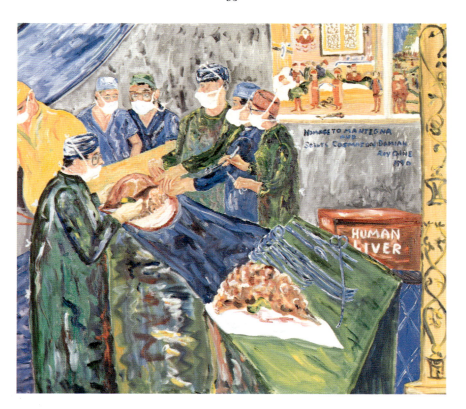

~86~

(85) A diptych by Mantegna in an antiphonal belonging to the Society of Antiquaries in London. The right-hand panel of the painting shows the removal of the leg from the corpse of a blackamoor, who had been buried recently. The main panel shows the recently completed operation. God is in the background, blessing the operation and ensuring its success. There are a number of inquisitive observers as well.

(86) This is my own tribute to Mantegna; a diptych, in oils, in which I show a motorcycle accident, the ambulance, the grieving parents, the Intensive Care nurse and the helicopter taking the liver to the hospital in the right-hand panel, whilst in the left-hand panel I have portrayed the operation taking place.

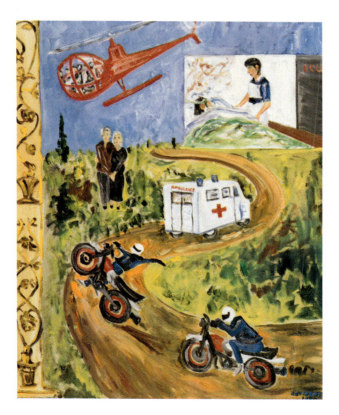

~86~

The scene was also depicted by Mantegna, in which the operation appears full of action. There is activity in the smaller panel of the diptych where the corpse of a blackamoor is exhumed, surrounded by a crowd of inquisitive bystanders. It is interesting, in the light of what followed in the modern era of transplantation that the medieval church regarded the idea of transplantation from a cadaver as a laudable and highly ethical procedure.

After painting a portrait of my patient, John Bellany, I realised that my perception of a patient was very different from the patient's self image. At this time, organ transplantation was a relatively new speciality; it had never been the subject matter of artists, apart from the medieval Saints, Cosmos and Damian. Over the past eight years, I have attempted to depict images of transplantation from the point of view of a surgeon; these include paintings of patients, colleagues, the operation, and the pioneers who have developed the science and surgery of transplantation. I have also depicted the surgical and anatomical features of some of the more complicated operations. In the course of trying to execute these images, I have formed friendships with patients, especially children, that previously would not have been possible due to time constraints and the traditional formal doctor/patient relationship. In the future, when organ transplantation is established as a routine and straightforward part of surgery, doctors will look back and wonder why we had so much trouble developing the technique. I hope that my paintings will go some way towards answering this question and capturing the disappointments and excitements of transplant surgery.

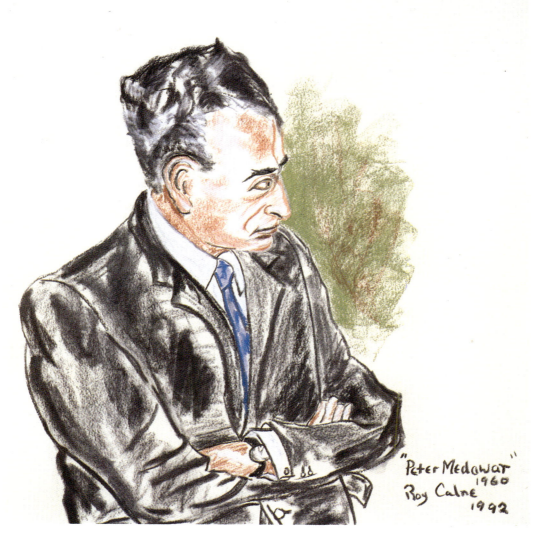

"Peter Medawar" 1960
Roy Calne 1992

~87~

CHAPTER SEVEN

(87) Sir Peter Medawar, the father of transplantation immunology. He was a tall and very handsome man, who listened to the comments of others and gave his advice and suggestions in a generous way. I am personally most grateful to him for his encouragement and friendship at the start of my training.

HISTORICAL BACKGROUND *to* ORGAN TRANSPLANTATION

In 1959 I became interested in the possibility of transplanting organs, however, there were two major hurdles to overcome before the technique could be used successfully. The first concerned the surgical procedure and the second was to discover ways of controlling the rejection of grafted organs. The biological process of rejection is still not fully understood and involves extremely important mechanisms in the body that are concerned with its defence against infection and cancer. The long lasting survival of a grafted organ requires a very delicate balance of the exact amount of immunosuppressive treatment, together with a great deal of good luck. As a result, the early organ grafting operations were extremely hazardous procedures with very few successes.

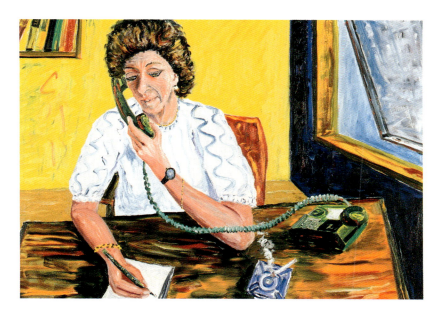

~88~

Celia Wight, our first Transplant Co-ordinator.

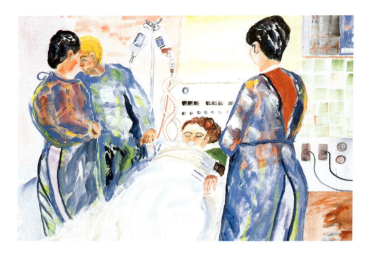

~89~

A drawing commissioned by the Spanish Co-ordinators Society, showing the training of co-ordinators and the management of this difficult and sensitive task.

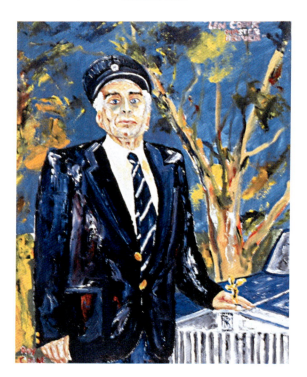

~90~

Mr Creek, who, for years, would drive our team to various hospitals in the UK to remove organs, and return them to Cambridge for transplantation.

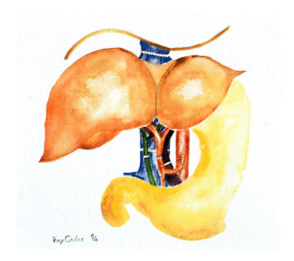

~91~

A schematic representation of a liver transplantation operation. The diagram shows the anastamoses of vena cava above and below the liver, as well as the hepatic artery, portal vein and bile duct.

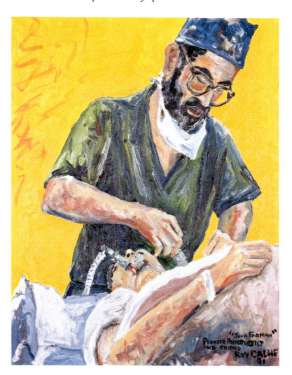

~92~

My colleague, Dr John Farman, an anaesthetist, who helped to establish liver transplantation in Cambridge. The skill of the anaesthetist has been an essential part in the development of this hazardous new form of surgery.

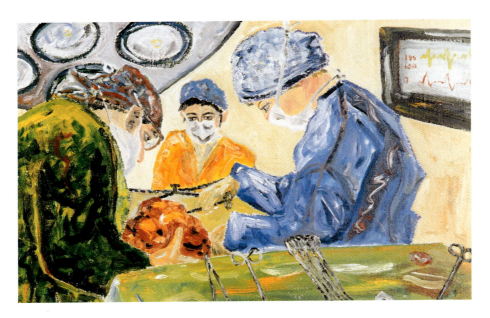

~93~

(93, 94, 95) The "moment of truth" in a liver transplant operation when the diseased liver has been removed and the new liver is about to be transplanted. At this point we do not know whether the operation is going to be successful or not. This illustration appeared on the cover of JAMA,[4] in which Dr Stephen Lock wrote:

"A Liver Transplant 1990" is a typical example of Calne's most recent clinical painting. Here he achieves a powerful sense of drama by allowing his half-length figures, contained within a pyramid, to occupy almost the entire pictorial space. The focal point is the removal of the diseased liver, to which the eye is drawn by the surgical instruments on the sludge-green table in the foreground. Instead of the bold contrasts of light and shadow favoured by the baroque artists to achieve a heightened effect, Calne here uses a diffuse, cold light - an appropriate choice for the clinical surroundings. His dramatic language is not one of line, but of colour; the vivid red of the diseased liver leaps out at the eye, contrasting with the cool blue figure on the right and with the surgeon himself. The viewer is reassured, though, by the atmosphere of calm, the concentration on the faces of the surgical team, and the capable hands at the centre of the drama.

Calne's present-day operating theatre, with its monitor screen, masked surgical team, and all the developments of modern technology, contrasts starkly with the arena in the latter half of the 19th century in which Thomas Eakins set his masterpiece the Gross Clinic (JAMA covers November 16 1964 and July 15 1983). No masks, gloves, or gowns here, but a surgical team in everyday clothes watched by a large audience — a thrilling drama dramatically lit, a blood-stained scalpel at its centre. What a long way surgery has come since then!"

[4]Journal of the American Medical Association, October 2, 1991 Vol. 266, No. 13

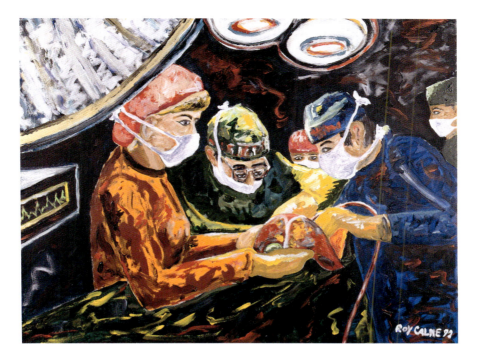

~94~

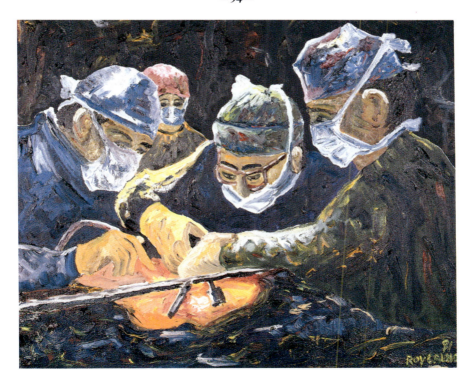

~95~

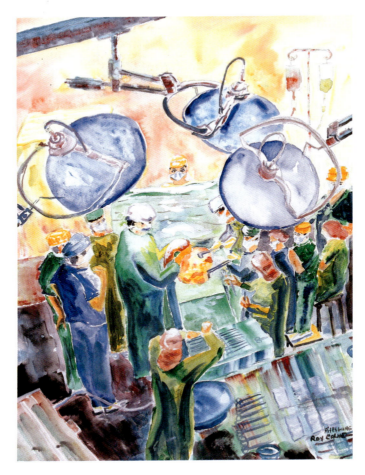

~96~

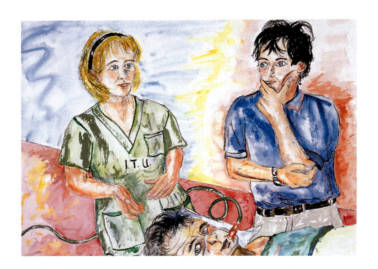

~97~

(96) A view of the Pittsburgh operating room from the observation dome. The operation in progress is being performed by Dr Tsakis.

(97) The Intensive Care Ward. The Sister and Consultant Anaesthetist are discussing the management of the patient, who seems to be well aware of the conversation.

(98) The HDU Sister who is responsible for the management of the patient after they have left the Intensive Care Unit.

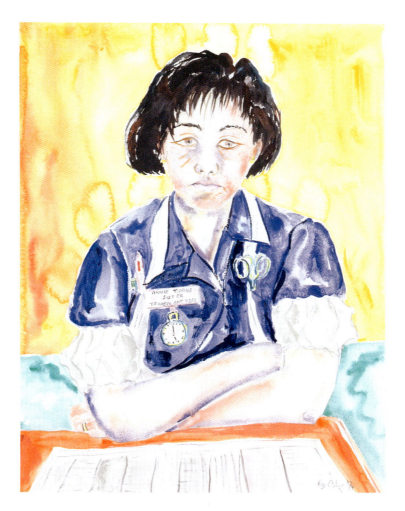

~98~

Surgery and Organ Preservation

In the 1950s, Dr Murray and his colleagues in Boston showed that kidney transplantation surgery could be successful, if the donor and recipient were a pair of identical twins. Identical twins are the same individual biologically and, therefore, grafts between identical twins cannot be rejected. The kidney is a suitable organ to transplant, since it is one of a pair, with a single artery, vein and urinary drainage tube, called the ureter.

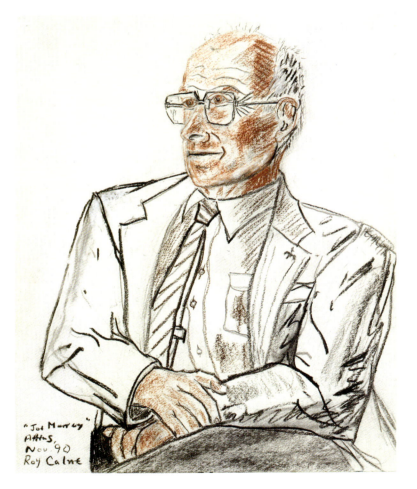

~99~

Dr Joseph Murray, pioneer transplant surgeon, who performed the first identical twin transplants. He demonstrated that if the operation was performed satisfactorily the patient could expect an excellent long-term result and received the Nobel Prize for his work.

Previously, the only treatment would have been recurrent dialysis with an artificial kidney machine, developed by the pioneer nephrologist, William Kolff, during World War II (1939-45) in Holland. The artificial kidney and appropriate surgical techniques for kidney transplantation made this the obvious first step in organ grafting. The usual technique, after removal of the kidney from its normal place in the loin, is to transfer it to the lower abdomen of the recipient, where it is partly protected by the pelvis. This is convenient for safe surgery and was first

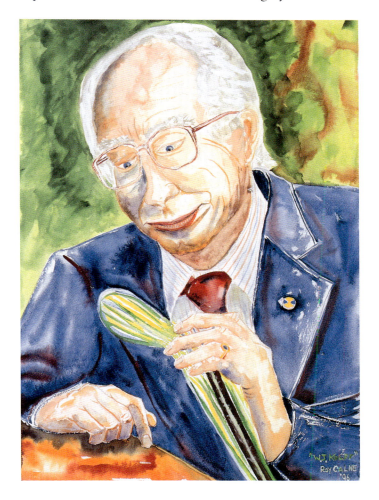

~100~

Dr William Kolff, who invented the first artificial kidney using cellophane and metal drums, during World War II. The artificial kidney has saved thousands of lives and was an essential step in the development of kidney transplantation. Dr Kolff has also pioneered the development of other artificial organs, notably the mechanical heart.

described by Dr René Kuss in Paris. The same technique was used by Dr Murray in Boston. Not only must the surgeon ensure that the joining of the blood vessels and ureter be done accurately, but speed is another element, since an organ deprived of its blood flow, which necessarily occurs during the transplant operation, rapidly deteriorates. It was found that cooling the kidney, by immersing it in cold innocuous fluid and

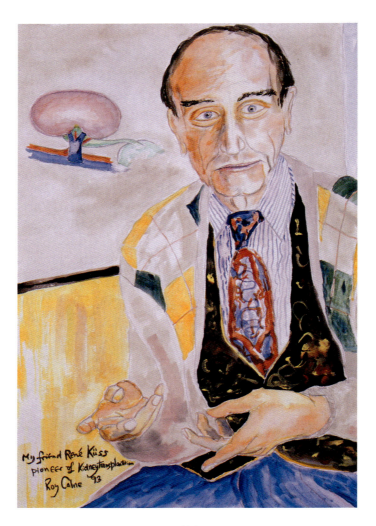

~*101*~

The French pioneer transplant surgeon, Dr René Kuss, who developed the pelvic extra-peritoneal approach for kidney transplantation. This technique was used by Dr Murray and has become a standard procedure. Dr Kuss performed some of the earliest kidney transplants in patients.

using a similar fluid to wash the blood out of it and cool it internally, greatly increased the period of time which the organ could be stored. In this way the organ could be transported in an icebox from one country to another and even between continents. One of the major pioneers in this field was Dr Belzer, who worked in California before becoming Professor of Surgery at the University of Madison, Wisconsin.

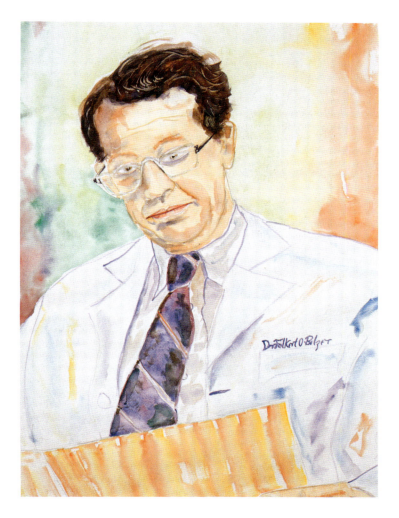

~102~

Dr Fred Belzer, Professor of Surgery at the University of Wisconsin. His life was devoted to organ transplantation and his research was concentrated on organ preservation.

Prior to Dr Murray's identical twin transplants, Dr David Hume, also at the Peter Bent Brigham Hospital in Boston, demonstrated that kidneys transplanted successfully, from a surgical point of view, would usually function for a short period of time and then be destroyed by rejection in a similar way to experimental kidney grafts and skin grafts. He found that sick patients dying of kidney disease sometimes suffered from an impaired immune system that resulted in the graft functioning much longer than expected. Hume was one of the great pioneers of transplantation, with a powerful intellect and enthusiastic good humour.

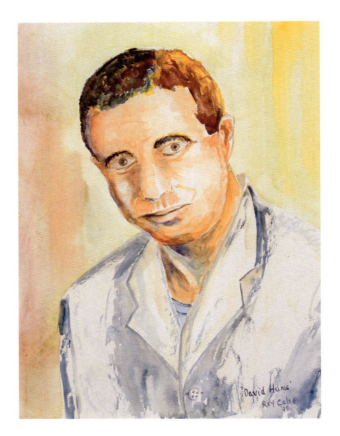

~103~

Dr David Hume, who performed the first successful non-twin transplants at the Peter Bent Brigham Hospital in Boston. Dr Hume later became Head of Surgery at the Medical College of Virginia. He was an outstanding intellect and leader in all aspects of organ transplantation. Sadly, he was killed in an aeroplane accident when he flew his light plane over the Rockies during bad weather.

It was not by accident that both Dr Murray and Dr Hume flourished in the department chaired by Dr Francis Moore, who was a distinguished pioneer in the study of human metabolism and the response of the body to surgery. He also started a programme of experimental liver grafting. He encouraged young surgeons with a friendly guiding hand and rigorous, but fair, constructive criticism and is the most impressive surgical professor I have encountered.

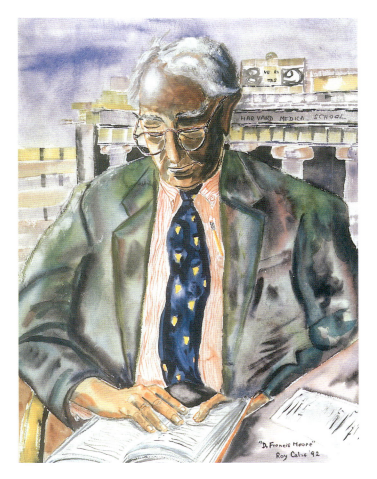

~104~

Dr Francis Moore, Surgeon-in-Chief at the Peter Bent Brigham Hospital. Dr Moore was a pioneer in liver transplantation and independently developed an experimental method of transplanting a liver in a dog at the same time as Dr Starzl was undertaking his research in Denver. Under Dr Moore's guidance, Dr Hume and Dr Murray were both able to pursue their pioneering transplant operations.

Transplantation Biology and Tolerance

The underlying science involved in graft rejection was discovered by Sir Peter Medawar and his colleagues. Medawar worked with the plastic surgeon, Tom Gibson, in the 1940s when there was a desperate need for skin grafts to treat burned servicemen. Medawar and Gibson studied skin grafts in rabbits and found that after the initial take the graft became infiltrated with inflammatory cells, such as lymphocytes and macrophages. The graft then became necrotic and turned into a scar. If the animal was then given another graft from the same donor, it was destroyed immediately without even a temporary take, whereas a graft from an animal unrelated to the original donor would be destroyed in the normal 'first set' manner. The rapid destruction of the 'second set' grafts was specific to the donor in question and demonstrated that graft rejection had similar features to other immune reactions. In the same way as we become immune to measles, having once suffered an attack, so we become immune to a specific individual's tissues after receiving a graft from that person. This biological process is part of the immune response, which has evolved to protect us from the invasion of bacteria and viruses and is also involved in surveillance and prevention of some cancers. If the immune system is destroyed, as happens, for example, in AIDS, the patient is vulnerable to infection from organisms that normally do not cause disease and is also susceptible to the development of cancers. To prevent rejection of a graft without paying the price of having one's immunity paralysed has been the chief stumbling block to the development of transplantation and failure to achieve this perfectly is still the cause of most disasters following organ grafting.

Medawar and his colleagues were asked if their observations might be of value in differentiating between identical and non-identical cattle twins. It was thought that skin grafting would rapidly settle this problem, but they were disappointed with the initial results. To their surprise, the grafts between non-identical cattle twins survived as well as those from identical twins. An explanation came from work by the Californian biologist, Ray Owen, who demonstrated that the circulation of the blood in the placentas of non-identical cattle twins is unusual, in that the blood mixes between the twins in the womb. This mixing results in both twins receiving red blood cells of different groups, which circulate harmoniously in their blood. The human equivalent would be an individual having some red cells of group A and some group B, a situation which has been described in non-identical twins by the British transplant pioneer Sir Michael Woodruff. Medawar believed that the unexpected findings in cattle twins may be due to this mixture of blood *in utero*.

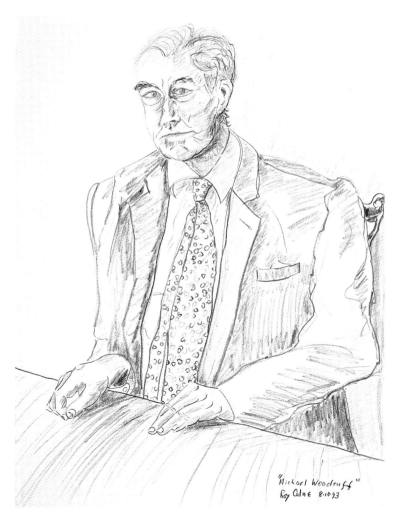

~105~

Sir Michael Woodruff was one of the early British transplant surgeons and immunologists. He was the first to describe the adaptation of grafts after transplantation. He and Waksman, independently produced the first anti-lymphocyte antibodies for the prevention of graft rejection.

He therefore decided to perform the definitive experiment, namely to inject cells from one strain of mouse into the embryo, or neonate, of another strain and then challenge it with a skin graft from the cell donor. This ground-breaking experiment was successful and showed that the developing immune system would accept foreign tissue as if it were its own. This phenomenon also occurred in chickens whose eggs were joined together, allowing the blood to be mixed between the embryos. Thus, Medawar had demonstrated that there was a means of overcoming rejection called "immunological tolerance". Unfortunately, the technique does not work after the neonatal period, and in some species, mid intra-uterine embryo life is already too late. Therefore, there is no direct clinical application of this procedure; nevertheless, it demonstrated that graft rejection could be prevented.

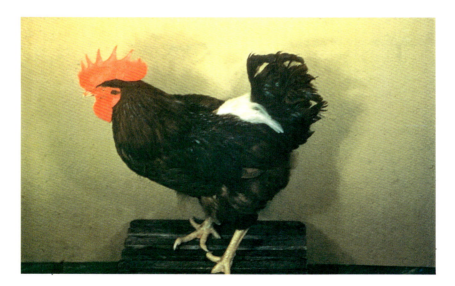

~106~

This illustration demonstrates a chicken with a white feather skin graft. This was one of the early experiments performed by Medawar and his colleagues, in which the developing chicken eggs were joined together by parabiosis. This slide was kindly given to me by Professor Leslie Brent.

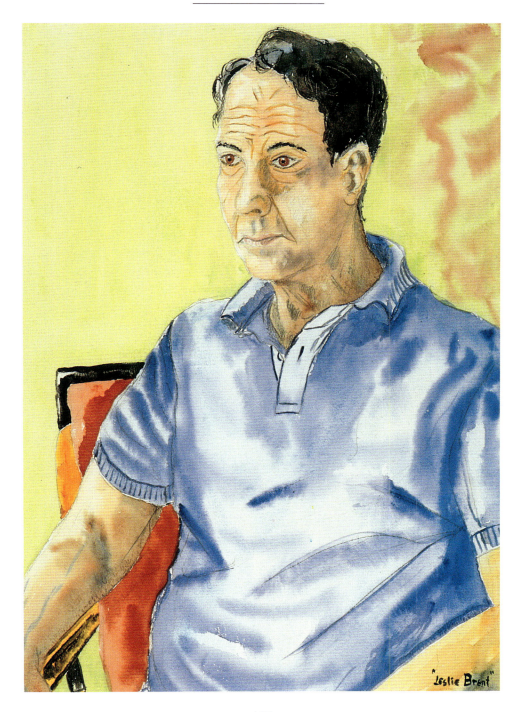

~107~

Leslie Brent was Professor of Immunology at St Mary's Hospital, London. The team of Brent, Dr Rupert Billingham, and Sir Peter Medawar demonstrated immunological tolerance.

The only harmful side effect, observed using this technique, was an immune "graft against host" disease, caused by the injected lymphocytes. Graft versus host disease is a very important complication in bone marrow transplantation. Medawar and his colleagues had found that injection of a potential donor's cells into an embryo, or a neonatal mouse or rat, caused the injected animal, after birth, to recognise and tolerate the donor's tissues as if they were its own. The imprint of the donor had, therefore, been incorporated into the "self product acceptance file" that we have for most of our own proteins. If someting goes wrong with this self acceptance, the stage is set for auto-immune disease.

Since the 1950s, tolerance has been the chief goal for those involved in clinical organ transplants. The surgical aspects of transplantation for a number of organs, including the kidney, liver, heart, lungs, and even the pancreas and intestines, have, to a large extent, been mastered. Methods of preserving each of these organs by cooling have been developed, but the biology of rejection remains a frustrating, unsolved hurdle, although we do have means of getting through or around the hurdles by use of tissue-typing and immunosuppressive drugs.

The first method used to prevent rejection involved destroying the immune system with X-irradiation and re-populating it with bone marrow from the donor. This is still the main principle of bone marrow transplantation, which is now established as a life saving treatment for many previously fatal diseases. In certain types of leukaemia the graft versus host disease may be advantageous, provided it is under control, because the grafted marrow may destroy the malignant leukaemic cells. Total body X-irradiation is too powerful and destructive for organ graft patients, who are usually already seriously ill: more gentle, yet effective methods had to be developed.

6-Mercaptopurine and Azathioprine

The use of the drug, azathioprine, as an immunosuppressant for solid organ grafts was a watershed in the development of clinical transplantation. In the Tuckahoe, New York laboratories of Burroughs Wellcome, Drs Hitchings and Elion started a programme of deliberate substitution of purines and pyrimidines to produce molecules that would act in a fraudulent manner to become incorporated in vital biological processes, but then poison the cells and prevent their division.

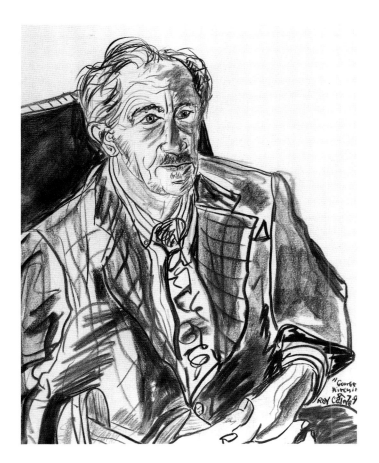

~108~

Dr George Hitchings, who together with Dr Trudy Elion (109), received the Nobel Prize for their work on the development of 6-mercaptopurine and azathioprine, which were the first drugs to be used in clinical immunosuppression. The agents were first developed for anti-cancer treatment and were part of a programme of synthetic purines and pyrimidines, which interfere with cell division.

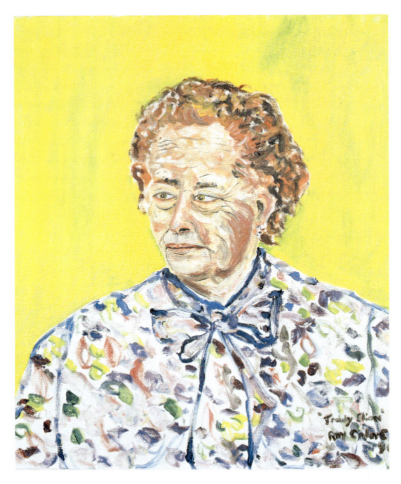

~109~

One of the agents, a thiopurine called 6-mercaptopurine, was recognised as a valuable tool in the therapy of certain leukaemias. Drs Schwartz and Damashek, working at Tufts Medical School in Boston, decided to use 6-mercaptopurine in experiments to inhibit the clonal proliferation of lymphocytes that occurs in response to an antigenic stimulus. In a paper in 1959, they showed that daily treatment of rabbits, challenged with a foreign protein, for two weeks with 6-mercaptopurine prevented the expected primary and later secondary response to that specific protein, but after the two week period of treatment the animals could react against other proteins. The two week course of 6-mercaptopurine appeared to have conferred a specific inhibition of antibody production, determined by the challenging protein at the commencement of the treatment. More important, however, was the observation that this effect lasted for a long time after the 6-mercaptopurine treatment had stopped. Thus, for a simple foreign protein antigen the drug 6-mercaptopurine was able to produce tolerance. At that time, the only clinically successful kidney transplants had been performed between identical twins and very closely matched sibling donors, who had been treated with total body X-irradiation. Many patients who received the same irradiation protocol, but with less well matched kidneys, developed uncontrollable rejection of the organs, or died from the side effects of the irradiation, infection being the major cause of death. Some clinicians persisted with this treatment, despite the almost universal failure; most agreed, however, that a safer, more effective form of immunosuppression was essential.

Following the publication of this work by Schwartz and Damashek, and in the hope of obtaining similar tolerance to organ grafts, I investigated the effect of this drug in dogs receiving renal allografts. I found that although 6-mercaptopurine did not produce immunological tolerance in dogs, it did prolong kidney graft survival. Similar observations were made independently by Zukoski and Hume. I wrote to Drs Hitchings and Elion at Burroughs Wellcome who had synthesised 6-mercaptopurine and asked if they had any better drugs. They were very interested in helping and suggested that I visit them in New York, on my way to begin a research fellowship in Dr Francis Moore's department, to work with Dr Murray. In 1960, arriving in New York by boat on the Queen Elizabeth, I took the little train to Tuckahoe and there Drs Hitchings and Elion generously provided me with a number of compounds that might be better than 6-mercaptopurine. They also started to cure my profound ignorance of the chemistry of the purines and pyrimidines. Following my visit to Tuckahoe, I studied the compounds given to me by Drs Hitchings and Elion in Dr Murray's laboratory and found an imidazolyl linked 6-mercaptopurine, later called azathioprine, was a little more effective and safer in preventing kidney graft rejection than 6-mercaptopurine itself.

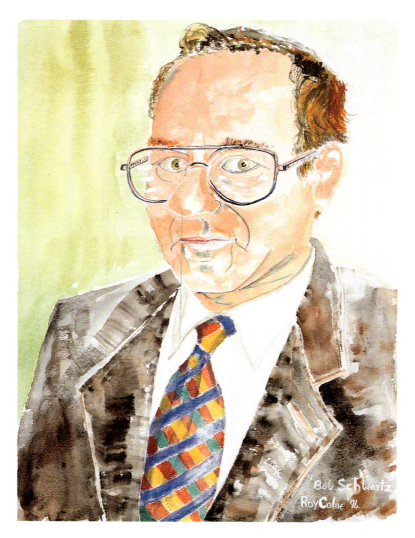

~*110*~

Dr Bob Schwartz, formerly a haematologist at Tufts University in Boston, and now book review editor for the New England Journal of Medicine. He worked with Dr Damashek and showed that 6-mercaptopurine, when administered to rabbits at the same time as a foreign protein would stop the animals producing antibodies to that protein. The animals were able to react against other different proteins. They called this effect "drug-induced immunological tolerance". On reading a paper on this subject, I decided to investigate the effect of 6-mercaptopurine in animals with kidney grafts.

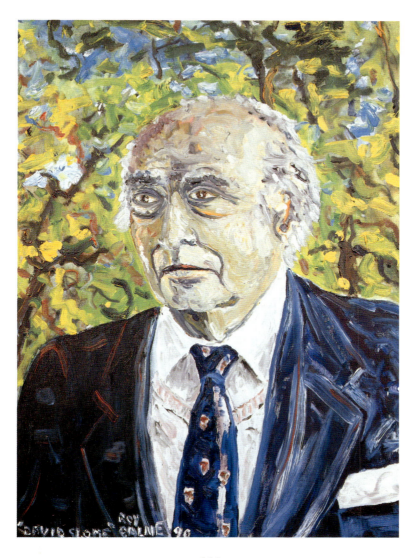

~111~

David Slome, Professor of Physiology at the Royal College of Surgeons of England. He allowed me to perform my first experiments involving kidney grafting in rats. Unfortunately, the experiments were not successful, but Professor Slome allowed me to attempt a kidney transplant in a dog instead. I had never seen this operation performed, but I was very fortunate since the first experiment was technically successful. Professor Slome continued teaching until he was nearly 90. He was a most extraordinarily generous man and a wonderful teacher and is remembered by thousands of surgeons who took their FRCS examination through the Royal College of Surgeons.

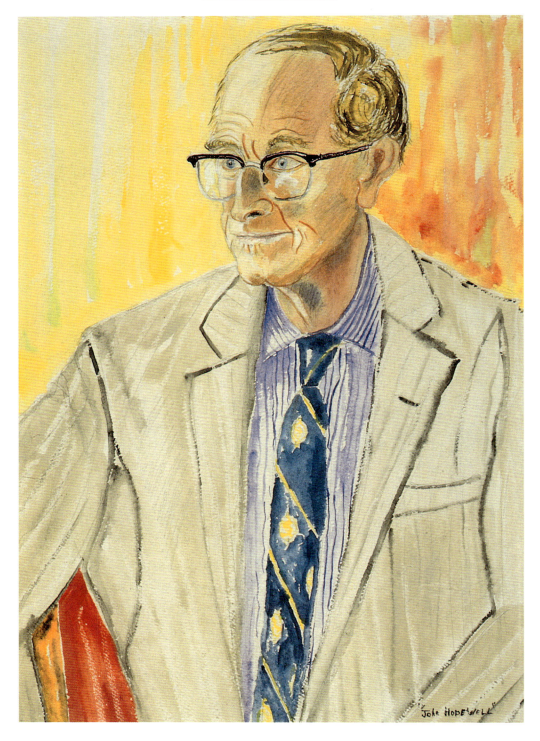

~112~

Mr John Hopewell, a Surgeon at the Royal Free Hospital, who encouraged me to undertake research into organ transplantation.

6-Mercaptopurine was the first of the thiopurines to be used in clinical transplants in England and France. Following the observations with azathioprine, a new protocol was inaugurated by Murray and his colleagues at the Peter Bent Brigham Hospital in 1962. The early results showed that azathioprine was a superior immunosuppressant to total body X-irradiation; however, it did not appear to be sufficiently effective alone for major clinical development. In 1960, Goodwin had demonstrated that an acute rejection crisis in a clinical renal transplant could be reversed by large doses of corticosteroids. In addition, corticosteroids in combination with azathioprine produced a drug protocol that gave promising results in renal allografts from donors that were not matched with the recipients. Working in Denver, Dr Starzl and his colleagues performed a series of renal allografts using azathioprine and corticosteroids for immunosuppression; their results were the best that had been produced so far in the clinic.

Rejection crises continued to occur and were treated with high doses of steroids, however, over-immunosuppression could lead to severe infection. There are a number of other specific side effects of azathioprine and steroids which could be very severe, particularly in children. For example, steroids stunt growth and cause Cushingoid facies, a disfiguring disease, which prevented the children from socialising normally. In addition, adults often developed aseptic hip necrosis. The chief side effect of azathioprine is bone marrow suppression and some patients suffer from liver damage. Despite these caveats, both azathioprine and steroids were used with success throughout the western world and Australasia and some of the early patients are still alive, thirty years after receiving renal allografts. This mode of immunosuppression was also used in transplants of the heart and liver, but would not permit transplantation of the lung or pancreas and the results of transplantation of liver and heart were poor.

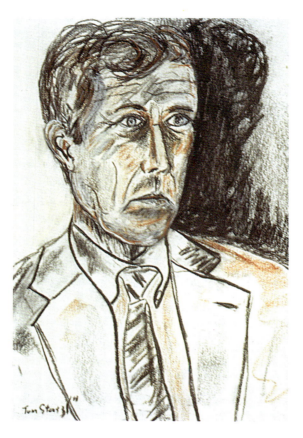

~113~

Dr Thomas Starzl, an extraordinary pioneer of organ transplantation, who started working on experimental liver transplantation in the late 1950s and early 1960s. He performed the first human liver transplant in 1963, having developed a very successful kidney transplant programme. He has pursued, with great enthusiasm, various areas of transplantation research and is still an active worker in this field. I sketched him in a churchyard in San Francisco the day before he had major cardiac surgery. He told me afterwards, that all the time he was posing he was suffering from a dreadful pain like a red hot poker through the middle of his body.

(114) Dr Jean Dausset, who received the Nobel Prize for his pioneering work on tissue-typing. He demonstrated that there was a special system of white cell groups, distinct from red blood cell groups, which were important in graft rejection.

Tissue-typing

The concept of individual specific proteins which act as antigens and cause an immune response to a graft was clarified by the work of Dausset and van Rood. The first practical method of tissue-typing depended on a technique of cytotoxicity introduced by Paul Terasaki, in which the cells killed by the antibody were recognised by their uptake of dye in a special tissue-typing tray. Tissue-typing of white cells is similar to red blood cell grouping. The major red blood cells are also important in organ grafting, since transgression of blood group rules usually results in the rapid destruction of a graft. The best results in kidney transplantation are obtained from family donors, particularly those matched for the major tissue-types. A perfect match occurs between 25% of siblings, and parents to child grafts are half-matched as are 50% of sibling donors.

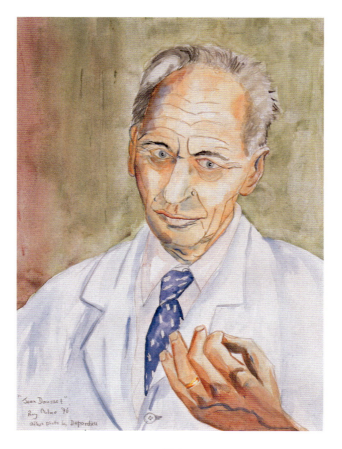

~114~

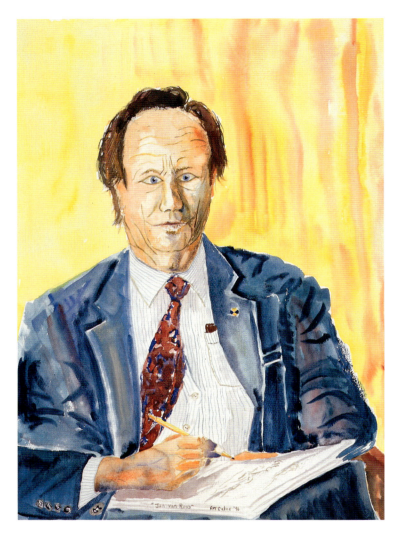

~115~

Dr Jon van Rood, another pioneer in tissue-typing and the first to use the technique in clinical bone marrow transplantation.

(116) Dr Paul Terasaki, a pioneer in tissue-typing, who developed the first practical cytotoxic test for tissue-typing, enabling laboratories to correlate their results, both nationally and internationally.

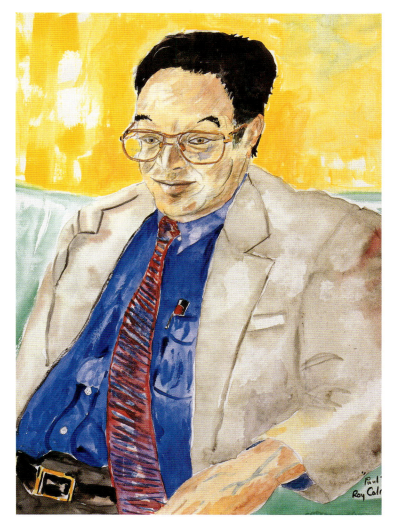

~116~

Anti-lymphocyte Antibodies

Over the next twenty years, efforts were made to find more efficient immunosuppressive drugs with less toxicity and more effect. The only useful agent produced was anti-lymphocyte serum, containing antibodies removed from the blood of animals, usually horses or rabbits, injected with human lymphocytes. The anti-lymphocyte serum preparations were sometimes effective and non-toxic, but batches varied; occasionally anti-lymphocyte serum produced severe serum sickness reactions, or did not seem to have any effect on the patient's lymphocytes.

Recently, much better anti-lymphocyte preparations are available and, the development of monoclonal antibodies has allowed the production of very specific antibodies each targeted against one molecule. These agents are now being studied and developed. In theory, monoclonal antibodies should be the best immunosuppressive agents because of the specific restriction of their action. They are most effective against lymphocytes circulating in the blood, but these only constitute 3% of the lymphocyte pool.

Cyclosporin

The next major advance in immunosuppression was the discovery of the immunosuppressive properties of a fungal peptide, cyclosporin, by the Swiss immunologist, Jean Borel, at Sandoz in Basel. Borel showed that cyclosporin would inhibit immune reactions in cultured cells and also prolong skin graft survival in mice. My colleagues and I studied the compound in animals with organ grafts and found it extremely powerful and effective. However, when we used it in the clinic we discovered that, although it was a better immunosuppressant than the combined azathioprine and steroids, it produced kidney damage, a side effect that we had not observed experimentally. This damage to the kidney could be minimised by administering small doses and combining cyclosporin with other drugs. The advent of cyclosporin changed the practice of transplantation worldwide. As a result, heart transplantation, pioneered by Norman Shumway and his research fellow, Richard Lower, in Stamford, was established as a major surgical technique. The first heart transplant in Man was performed by Christian Barnard in 1967, but it was only after cyclosporin was available that heart transplantation results became sufficiently good to be practiced widely, and for the first time lungs and the pancreas could be transplanted successfully. The pancreas is often transplanted together with a kidney for patients with diabetic renal failure, and recently the intestine has been transplanted in patients who have lost function of the small bowel. Sometimes other organs are transplanted together with the intestine, for example, the liver, since intravenous feeding for patients without bowel function can damage the liver.

~117~

Dr Jean Borel, who discovered the immunological properties of cyclosporin. He demonstrated that the drug was a powerful immunosuppressant both in vitro and in vivo and that it would prolong skin grafts in mice. The use of this drug in clinical transplantation marked a watershed in the development of organ transplantation, turning it from a dangerous and largely experimental procedure, to the most effective form of therapy for many diseases.

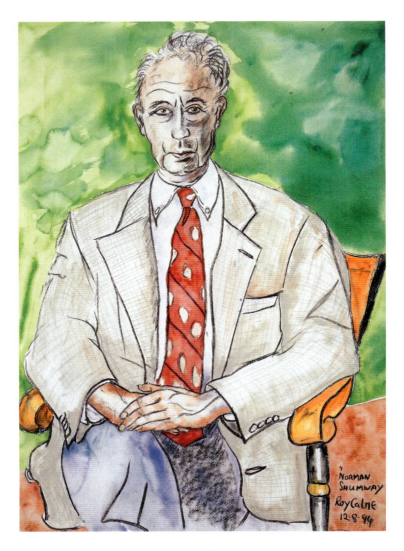

~118~

Dr Norman Shumway who, together with Dr Lower, in Stanford, developed a safe method of heart transplantation in the dog. The procedure was later performed in Man by Dr Christian Barnard. Norman Shumway's pioneering efforts have often been overshadowed by the media's early accounts of Christian Barnard's achievements. Barnard was the first person who had the courage and the facilities to perform a heart transplant in Man.

The Liver Effect

My own interest moved from the kidney to the liver. My fascination lay in the unique immunological features of liver grafting in the pig and the rat, where the liver transplants sometimes survive indefinitely without rejection in animals given no immunosuppressive treatment. Liver immunosuppression is powerful and we have spent many years trying to understand the mechanisms and its application in surgery. It is of interest that a liver transplanted at the same time as a kidney, from the same donor, protects the kidney from rejection. The same is true for other organs transplanted together with the liver. The first human liver transplant was performed by Dr Thomas Starzl in 1963. The

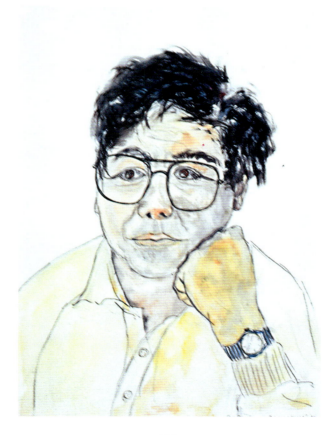

~119~

My colleague, Dr Kamada, who worked with me in Cambridge for nine years and researched the immunoprotective effect of the liver. The microsurgical techniques of Dr Kamada allowed analysis of this phenomenon in rats.

operation was a huge procedure in patients usually moribund and the early results were bad. The liver is often rejected in Man and some patients develop sepsis or recurrence of their original disease, particularly if they suffered from cancer or hepatitis due to a viral infection. Since we had established a satisfactory experimental technique for liver grafting through our immuno-logical studies in the pig, I started a programme of liver trans-plantation in Cambridge in 1968. I was very fortunate in having Dr Francis Moore visiting from the Peter Bent Brigham Hospital. He had independently pioneered experimental liver transplantation at the same time as Dr Starzl. He assisted and gave strong moral support at the first liver transplant in Europe. As with any new procedure there is always opposition from col-leagues, but the authority and eloquent advocacy of Dr Moore,

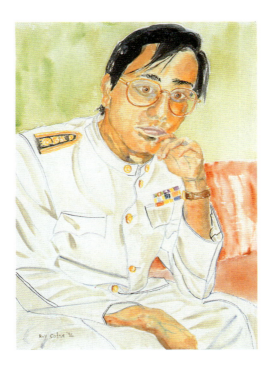

~120~

Dr Voravit Sriwatanawongsa from Thailand who examined the liver effect, using the extremely difficult microsurgical technique of re-transplanting a liver graft after the bone marrow-derived cells in the liver had changed from those of the donor to recipient-type. His studies were very important in helping to understand this phenomenon.

trying to help patients for whom there was no other treatment, helped to launch liver transplantation in our hospital.

Since the introduction of cyclosporin in the late 1970s, organ transplantation has become a major part of surgery in all developed countries. Increasingly ambitious transplants have been performed in the very young, the elderly, or involving multiple organs transplanted at the same time. We have also performed a small number of combined heart, lungs and liver transplants. The first patient was particularly memorable; she was referred for a liver transplant operation, but was too sick to undergo surgery, due to a severe lung disease requiring continuous oxygen treatment. She requested that something was done and we told her that she would need a heart, lungs and liver, and that had never been done before. She said well, that would do nicely

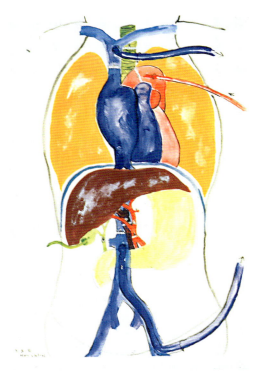

~121~

Diagram of a heart-lung bypass circuit that we used in a combined heart, lungs and liver transplant in collaboration with our colleagues at Papworth Hospital.

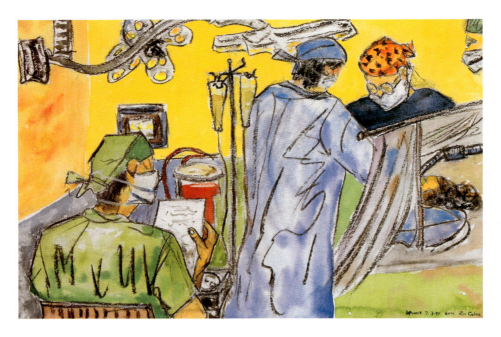

~122~

An impression of heart, lungs and liver transplantation in progress, sketched in the operating room.

and so, in collaboration with our colleagues in Papworth Hospital, the operation was performed and the patient has had an extremely smooth post-operative course, living as a busy housewife, well ten years after operation.

In the event of kidney graft failure, the patient can be maintained in reasonable health by recurrent dialysis, either of the blood or the peritoneal cavity. For liver and heart disease there is no such luxury available; although a heart-lung machine will maintain a patient during a surgical operation, attempts at implanting artificial hearts have been disappointing. There is no substitute for the liver, since it is the main metabolic factory of the body, synthesising proteins, removing toxic substances from the blood, and secreting bile to aid digestion. For a patient who has rejected a liver graft, or if the liver has failed for other reasons, the only treatment is a repeat liver transplant. A few patients have required three or four repeat transplants and it amazes me that a patient who has been through such a terrible operation can be prepared to accept, or actively request, another liver transplant.

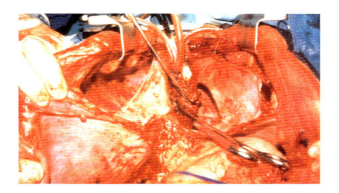

~123~

The empty body cavity after removal of the heart, lungs and liver.

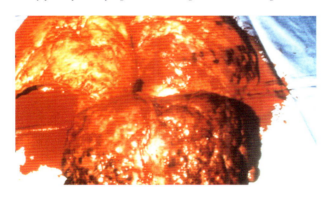

~124~

The lungs and liver after removal. The heart was not diseased and was used as a donor organ for another patient, the so-called "domino procedure".

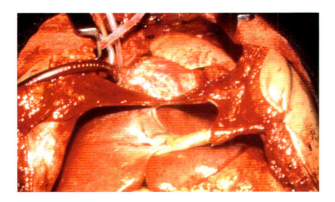

~125~

The donor organs transplanted and reperfused; the liver is below, the heart in the middle and the lungs on each side.

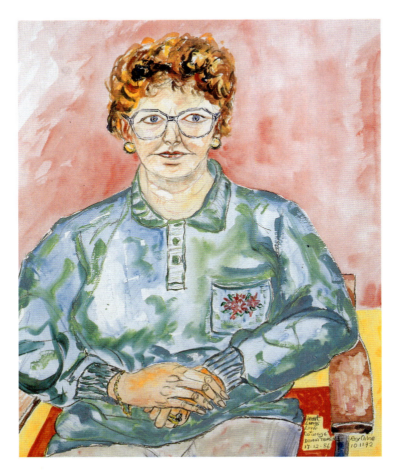

~126~

This is the first patient ever to receive a heart, lungs and liver transplant. She
is an active housewife and is still well, ten years after surgery.

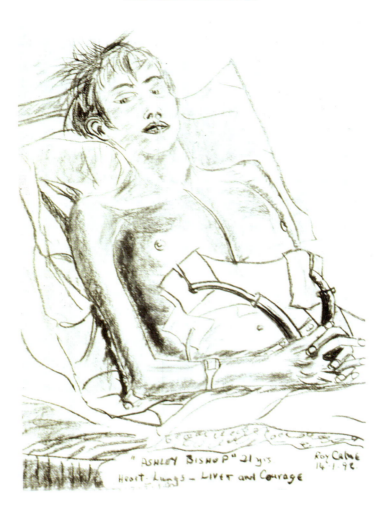

"ASHLEY BISHOP" 21 yrs   Roy Calne
14-1-9?
Heart-Lungs - LIVER and Courage

~127~

Another patient who had a heart, lungs and liver transplant. After the
portrait was completed he asked to see it and gave me a big smile. I
asked him why he was smiling and he said it was the first time he had
ever seen air fill his lungs. Sadly he developed an infection from
which he succumbed a few weeks after the operation.

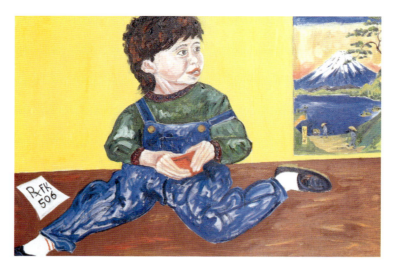

~*128*~

The first child in Europe to be treated with the new immunosuppressant, FK506 or "Prograf". This child had developed the symptoms of graft rejection, but had failed to respond to corticosteroids and anti-lymphocyte serum. His liver function rapidly improved when he was administered FK506.

Current Developments

There are now two new immunosuppressive drugs registered, FK506 or "Prograf", and mycophenolate mofetil or "Cellcept". The former is effective in minute doses and acts in a similar manner to cyclosporin, although it has a completely different chemical structure. In contrast, Cellcept is an anti-proliferative drug, which has a similar action to azathioprine, but appears to be more powerful in inhibiting rejection.

When cyclosporin was introduced into clinical organ transplantation it was used alone, or in combination with corticosteroids. Later, it was combined with azathioprine as a triple drug regimen. In some centres, polyclonal or monoclonal anti-lymphocyte antibodies, were given together with the three drugs. To treat a patient with four different immunosuppressive agents requires very careful clinical monitoring. There are many hazards, including, over-immunosuppression causing infection and the danger of malignancy, particularly B-cell lymphomas. The exact immunosuppressive protocol followed by different centres varies in detail, but for the past decade, triple therapy with cyclosporin, azathioprine and steroids has been the most common form of treatment. In the next decade the new drugs will be incorporated into a variety of protocols, the management of which will require great skill.

Where Do the Grafts Come From?

Since the kidney is a paired organ, live donation is possible. The best results are obtained in transplants between identical twins with the next best occurring between patients who are closely related and a good tissue-type match. The ordinary red blood cell groups are also important and need to be compatible for organ transplants. In addition, there is a whole system of tissue-type antigens, called human lymphocyte antigens (HLA), part of the major histocompatibility complex (MHC), which has now been genetically defined and resides in a complicated DNA formation on the sixth human chromosome. Tissue-typing using the polymerase chain reaction (PCR) is extremely accurate and is now performed as a routine laboratory procedure. The purpose of the tissue antigens is to facilitate the recognition of foreign antigens and the diversity of human tissue-types has profound biological significance, but it is not helpful to the transplant surgeon and his patients. Following pregnancy, blood transfusion or graft rejection patients may develop antibodies. A check for destructive antibodies, called a "cross match", is always made between the patient's serum and the potential donor's white blood cells. A positive cross match means that the grafting operation should not go ahead. Excluding the cross match, the importance of tissue-typing outside the family has been frequently debated, since powerful immunosuppression can often overcome tissue type incompatibilities. There is, however, no doubt that a graft will do better the closer the match of donor and recipient.

Due to the shortage of organs, live donors have also been used to provide lobes of liver and lung. The operations are much more hazardous and there have been fatalities in donors. However, where there is no other option, parent to child transplantation would seem to be ethically justified. If there is no suitable, living, related donor, which is the case for most potential recipients of organ grafts, then removal of an organ from a dead person is the next best option and, of course, this is necessary for most heart and liver transplants. Patients who die from cancer or infection are unsuitable as cadaver donors, since the fatal disease in the donor is likely to be transferred to the recipient *via* the graft. Most suitable donors are therefore the victims of road traffic accidents and brain haemorrhage. It is essential to remove the donor organ quickly after death; in western countries the usual practice is to remove the organs from patients who have brain stem destruction, but have their ventilation maintained artificially by a machine. In this way, the organ can be removed without it suffering any initial damage through cutting its blood supply.

Clearly, the issues of organ donation raise ethical dilemmas, as does the selection of recipients and the arrangement of priority lists for organ transplantation. To give priority to patients who are the most ill may produce poor overall results and block expensive Intensive Care beds, denying treatment for other patients who may fare much better. The health profession, governments and ethicists have agonised over these concerns and I will discuss some of them in the next section.

Organs from Animals?

The improved results of organ transplantation have highlighted the ever present shortage of suitable donor organs for patients who might benefit from a transplant. In the United Kingdom, over the past thirty years, there has been little change in the number of people willing to donate an organ after death. Between 25 and 30% of the population have consistently been opposed to organ donation for themselves, or their relatives, whilst it must be admitted that most of these individuals, if they need a transplant, will change their minds completely on this issue.

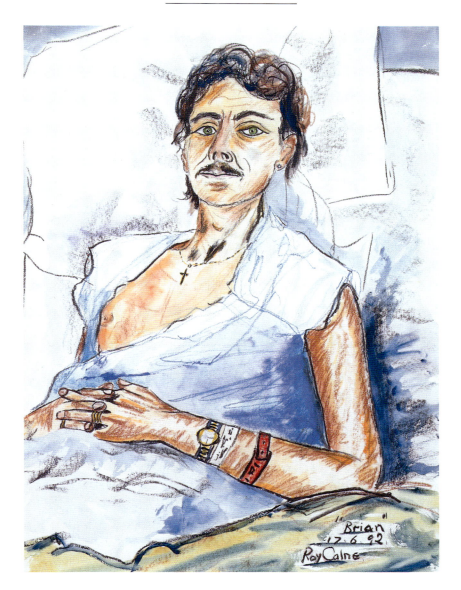

~129~

A patient in Pittsburgh, waiting for a liver transplant from a baboon. He was a very courageous man, who explained to me that he expected the operation to be successful, but if it was not, he hoped that the doctors would gain valuable information that would help other patients in the future. He asked me to paint the colour of his eyes correctly, they were green.

Since the waiting list for organ transplants steadily increases year by year, there is mounting pressure to study xenotransplantation and overcome the barriers that exist in grafting organs from animals to Man. Early attempts at xenotransplantation from primate species to Man failed, although one patient experienced some success with a chimpanzee kidney graft for nine months. However, there are contraindications to organ donation from primates since chimpanzees are an endangered species and other primates are phylogenetically more distant to Man. An exaggerated form of organ rejection, called concordant xenograft rejection, is observed in such cases. Rejection between widely different species is usually immediate due to naturally occurring antibodies, called a discordant reaction.

Many scientists believe that the pig would be an attractive species as an organ donor, since breeding colonies could be easily established with no threat to the species. In addition, the pig has high parity, breeds well, grows rapidly to a convenient size and is cared for relatively easily. Although the idea may still be distasteful to some, it is hard to see how the majority of people in a meat-eating society could object to this plan on moral or ethical grounds. Pigs are already used to provide society with other medical materials, and the use of porcine insulin, or porcine heart valves, has been embraced with enthusiasm because of the benefits offered to patients. From a surgical point of view, organs of the appropriate size can be obtained from pigs to transplant into patients. Although pig and human physiology may be similar, there are important differences between the two species that have resulted from a divergence in evolution of some 400 million years. Thus, virtually every protein produced by the pig is different, to a greater or lesser extent, from the equivalent human protein. The natural life span of the pig is fifteen years and we do not know yet whether organs would be able to function for longer if rejection could be prevented.

In the Department of Surgery at Cambridge University, David White has studied complement and complement activation in the xenograft reaction. It would seem that if complement activation can be prevented, *via* both the direct and indirect pathways, then hyper-acute discordant rejection should not occur. Complement present in the blood stream is normally maintained in an inactive form by species-specific complement regulators. Encouraging results have been achieved through introducing the human complement regulator, Decay Accelerating Factor (DAF), into pig embryos. The success of this transgenic technique has provided both hetero[5]- and homozygote[6] transgenic animals, expressing human DAF, whose organs do not undergo hyper-acute rejection when transplanted into primates. This is an important first step in understanding and overcoming the xenograft reaction. Having prevented the hyper-acute rejection, a destructive immunological reaction against the graft can only be curtailed by high doses of immunosuppressive drugs and long-term survival has not yet been achieved.

There have been considerable concerns expressed that xenografting could activate animal viruses and prions, which could be a hazard, not only to the patient in question, but might spread to non-transplanted individuals. It has been suggested that the HIV virus originally came from wild primates and that the prion disease Bovine Spongiform Encephalitis (BSE) may have been modified from the scrapie virus in sheep *via* cattle to become pathogenic to Man.

The government in the UK plans to regulate xenografting by imposing a careful scrutiny on its development. This will ensure that human trials are undertaken in a responsible manner, with special safeguards to minimise any danger to patients and the rest of the community. Work on xenografting continues with ever-increasing momentum and one can anticipate advances in this field that would be a boon to many sick patients if they could be offered therapeutically valuable xenografts.

---

[5]heterozygote transgenic animals – one of the pair of chromosomes expresses DAF

[6]homozygote transgenic animals – both of the pair of chromosomes expresses DAF

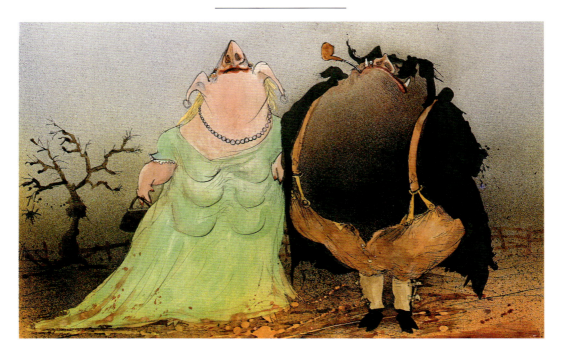

~130~

An illustration by the distinguished artist, Ralph Steadman, from the new edition of Orwell's,
Animal Farm . The illustration shows "Napoleon" and his lady going to have supper with the farmers.
In this satirical novel, the pigs became more and more like humans without the benefit of any
transgenic techniques.

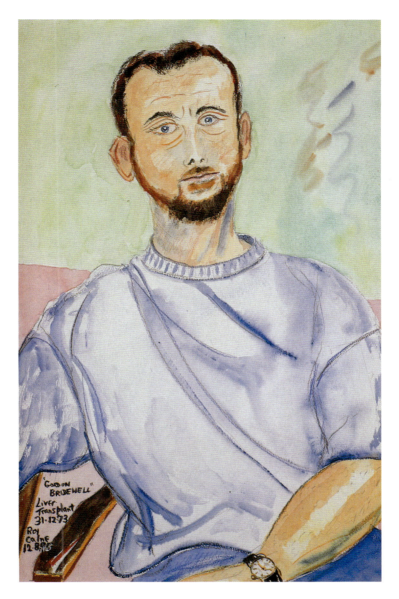

CHAPTER EIGHT

(131) Gordon Bridewell, 22 years after he received a liver transplant and still working as a vehicle engineer. He is a most remarkable patient; in his 20's, he came to us with a huge malignant tumour of the liver and the rest of his liver was cirrhotic, due to a hepatitis B infection. It is doubtful whether Mr Bridewell would now be offered this operation, since both of these conditons are contraindications to liver transplantation. However, he recovered from his operation and has excellent liver funct:on 22 years later.

PATIENTS, NURSES, DOCTORS, DONORS *and* SCIENTISTS

The story of transplantation is a saga of hope, excitement, disappointment, misery and elation. In just forty years, transplantation has moved from a biological concept, shrouded in mystery, to a practical and much sought after form of treatment. While the surgery is well established, much of the biological mystery still remains. The essential players in the development of transplantation were those doctors, nurses and scientists who believed that the endeavour was worthwhile and would one day succeed. Praise must also go to the patients, who, faced with inevitable deterioration of their quality of life and certain death, were prepared to take a risk which might incur further pain, discomfort and disappointment. Lastly, we should remember the relatives of those who had suffered fatal accidents, and others who had volunteered, and sometimes insisted that, one of their organs should be used to try and help a loved one. The repetitive chorus 'It can't be done, it shouldn't be done, it won't ever succeed' has acted as a stimulus to the believers that they would disprove the establishment view.

New ideas are seldom welcomed by those in authority and this applies in other fields, not just transplantation. Machiavelli wrote:

"There is nothing more difficult to take in hand, more perilous to conduct, or more uncertain in its success than the introduction of a new order of things, because the innovator has for enemies all those who have done well under the old conditions and lukewarm defenders in those who may do well under the new."

In the early development stages of organ transplantation, the concept was not in general accepted by the profession, it was regarded as an experimental procedure indulged in by a small number of innovative surgeons. The early opposition to our new form of treatment was replaced when there are some successes

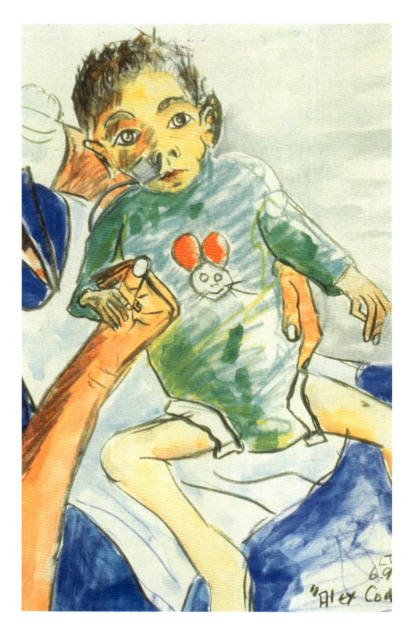

~132~

The youngest child referred to us for a liver transplant. At six weeks old he was
so wasted and sick that he required more than a month of intravenous feeding
before he was well enough to receive his liver transplant.

by the feeling, 'oh well, this is a one-off lucky chance, one swallow doesn't make a summer'. But in fact, in medical progress one swallow is the harbinger of a summer, the fact that it can be done spurs research workers to greater and more intense efforts, often culminating in a high level of success with important details previously not readily appreciated becoming part of a routine.

The operation of liver grafting required vast resources and huge volumes of blood, that often exhausted the local blood bank. We now perform two liver transplants a week and it is regarded as a routine procedure, requiring very small volumes of blood. Following the introduction of cyclosporin, results improved and the applications of grafting techniques increased. Once established, the voices of opposition changed to a clamour for more transplant centres, more donors and increased access for patients who might benefit from this form of treatment. Very often, the pioneers who were derided by the establishment are forgotten.

Children are particularly difficult patients, from the ethical point of view, and also in their care and management. A child under the age of two is not able to understand the need for an operation and, therefore, the discussion must centre on the parents and their wishes. An older child with liver disease is usually vulnerable due to the length of time the child will have spent in hospital and the repeated unpleasant tests, medicines and invasive procedures. These children are usually terrified of doctors and nurses, but I have found that if I have time to sit down with pencil and paper, I can communicate with the child and try to allay some of their fears. In fact, the whole procedure may be quite fun and the child will sometimes draw me at the same time. Having finished a drawing, I usually give a photocopy to the child to colour in. In this way, it is possible to be friends with the child and not be intimidating.

I have tried to record, using drawings and paintings, some of the stages in the development of transplant surgery, and, in particular, the courage of the patients, the hopes of their relatives and the generosity of donors.

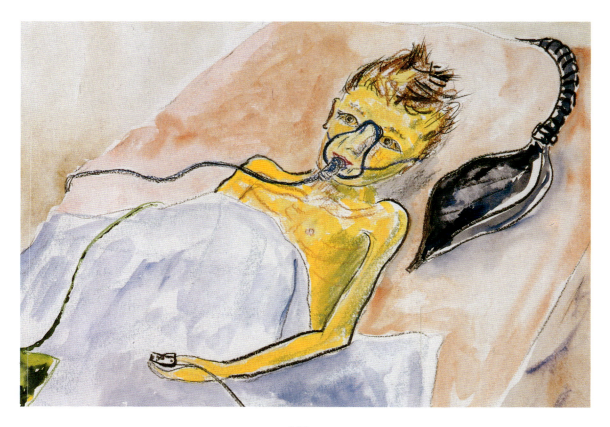

~*133*~

A child with congenital immuno-deficiency disease, not associated with HIV. Sadly, he never fully recovered after the operation and developed a fatal lung infection some weeks later.

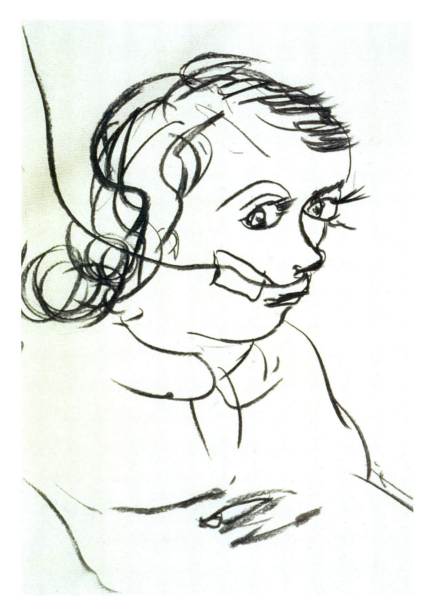

~134a~

A rapid sketch of a child who has spent most of her life in hospital and who
is suspicious of doctors and nurses. She has extraordinarily long eyelashes,
which look beautiful, but are part of her chronic illness.

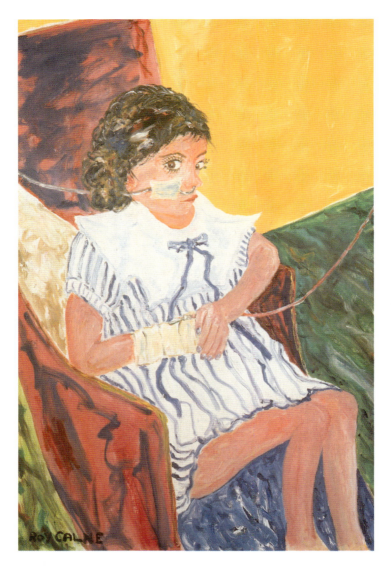

~134b~

An oil painting based on the previous sketch. This was reproduced on the front cover of the Journal of the American Medical Association[7], September 23/30 1992, in which Dr Therese Southgate commented as follows:

"Child After a Liver Transplant" was painted in 1989 by the surgeon, it nevertheless expresses the child's point of view. The large expanse of green, juxtaposed against an equally large expanse of red, attests to the violence implicit in the procedure. Tastefully out of sight, explicit violence nevertheless exists, say the colours. Not only the obvious violation of the body of the patient, necessitated by the surgical procedure, but the violence to the sensibilities of surgeon and team — and, lest one forgets, to the donor, who probably died a sudden and untimely death.

The large expanse of yellow wall, reminiscent of the yellow van Gogh used, suggests the overwhelming anxiety felt by the patient. The patient, meanwhile, at a time when the individuality of even her immune system must be suppressed, is painted in a colour, from hair, to dress, to fingernails, that sharply distinguishes her from her background. But the real feeling of the painting is in the figure of the child: her knees together, her eyes large, the eyelashes prominent, but with a glance that, while not altogether open, is not an outright refusal. She is willing, but wary, young, but old, innocence prematurely lost……..."

[7]Journal of the American Medical Association, September 23–30, 1992, vol. 268, No. 12

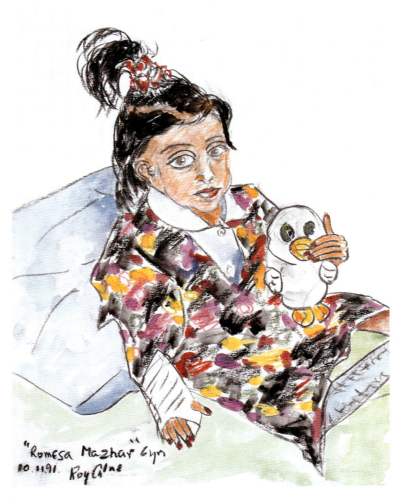

~135~

Another child after a liver transplant, clutching her baby duck.

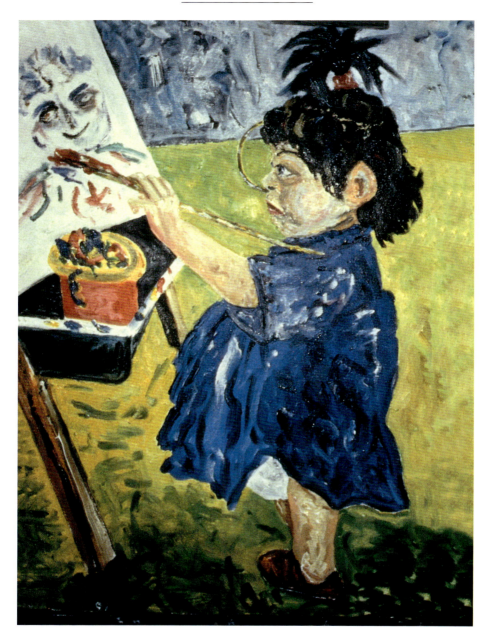

~136~

This child eventually had four liver transplants. She was full of life and spirit and came from the city of Belfast, where this painting now hangs in the Children's Hospital. She rejected one liver after another, and suffered grievously. However, her spirit was an inspiration to other parents and she was an exceedingly popular patient in the children's ward.

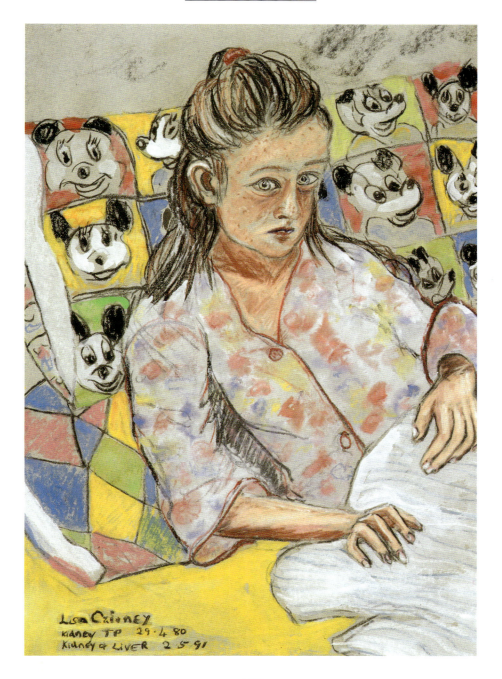

~137~

A child with oxalosis, whose brother had the same condition. Both children were treated with combined liver and kidney transplants and both suffered complications which required further transplant operations.

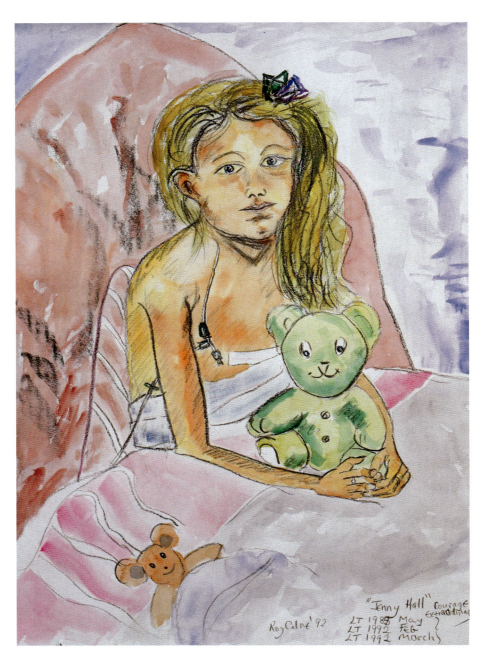

~138~

This child was also the recipient of more than one liver transplant; she is shown here recovering from the operation.

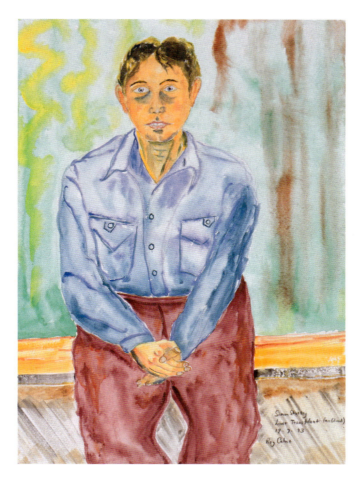

~139~

This young boy belonged to a family of devout Jehovah's Witnesses. The parents were willing to allow their child to receive a liver transplant, but they asked if I would perform the operation without a blood transfusion, since this was against their religion. They had already been to a number of transplant centres, but they had been unable to find a surgeon who was prepared to operate without the use of blood. I explained to the parents that, whatever their beliefs, it was not fair to the whole team to undertake an operation where success might be turned to failure, just for the want of one unit of blood. I explained to them that I would try to perform the operation without the use of blood, but I would require their permission to give blood if the situation became a matter of life and death. Reluctantly they accepted this arrangement. However, the parents wishes were fulfilled and the operation was perfomed without a single unit of blood. Every year they send me a card thanking me for adhering to their wishes and giving me an update on their son's progress.

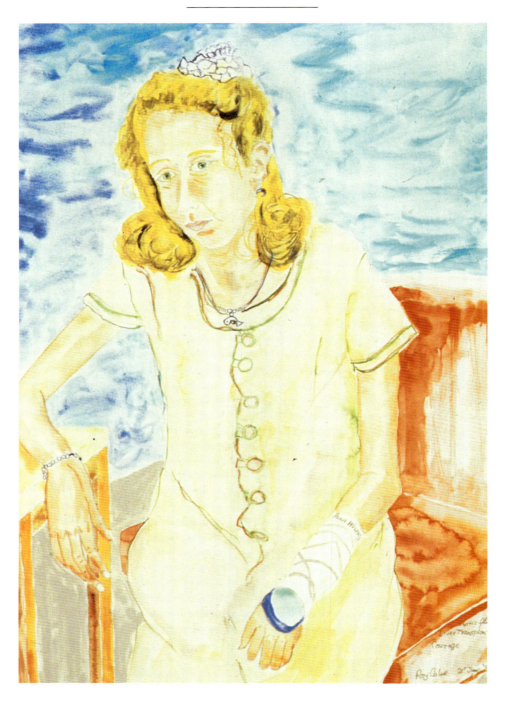

~140~

A young teenager with cystic fibrosis, recovering from her liver transplant. She is a very interesting girl who told me that the disease was of enormous consequence to her whole family, friends and their way of life.

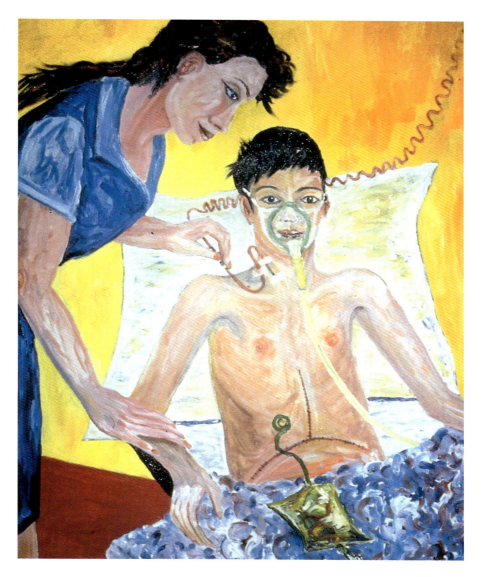

~141~

Young child being tended by a nurse after his liver transplant. He was old enough to understand the purpose of this painful and distressing operation and appreciated the devoted care of his nurse.

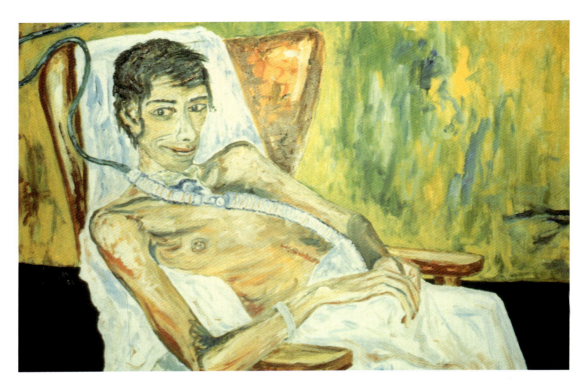

~142~

This boy had Wilson's disease and had lapsed into terminal coma, so it was not possible to speak to him before the operation. He was in a desperate state after surgery and required a tracheotomy and mechanical ventilation. He was, however, a very cheerful and optimistic lad who was about to go to university. Sadly, he developed a lung infection from which he died some weeks later. His parents wished to see my portrait of him, but my wife and I were worried that it would upset them. However, it had the opposite effect; they felt that this was a tribute to their son's courage and they requested a reproduction.

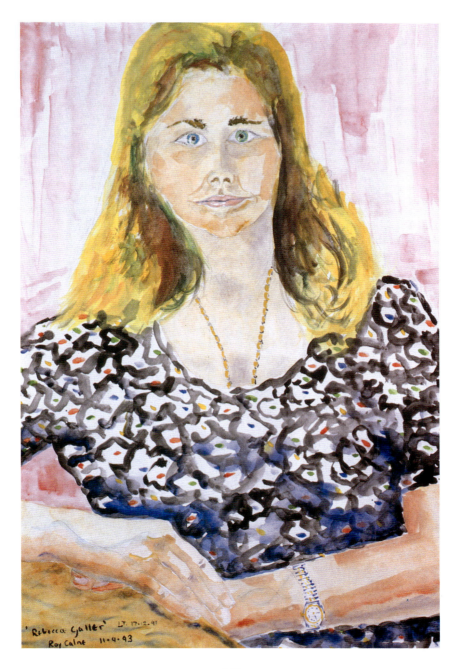

~*143*~

This painting shows Rebecca Galler, who made a full recovery after a liver transplant and has devoted much energy and effort to raising public awareness towards liver transplantation. When I met her in Washington, where I painted this portrait, she was one of the active members of the organisation TRIO (Transplantation Recipients International Organisation).

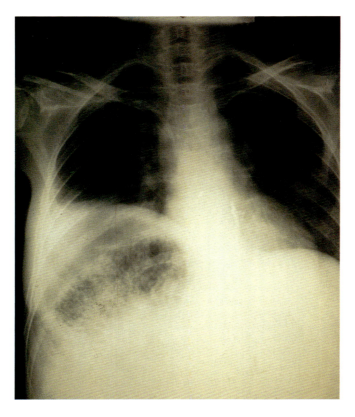

~144~

(144, 145, 146,) These three paintings portray, Eileen O'Shea, who worked as a nurse, and underwent four liver transplant operations. On the tenth day after her first transplant her recovery was suddenly reversed and she entered a state of extreme shock. A chest X-ray showed what appeared to be a lung under the diaphragm, but which was actually the liver, infected with gas gangrene, an extremely unusual and dangerous condition. We immediately removed the liver and performed a porta-caval shunt, since we did not have another donor organ. We contacted our colleagues in the UK, but there were no suitable livers available. Fortunately, a team led by Professor Pichlmayer in Hanover, were removing a liver for one of their patients. They very generously sent the liver to Cambridge, which we transplanted 24 hours later, therefore saving the life of our patient. However, the liver was the wrong blood group and was rapidly rejected. Later, she received a third liver and whilst she was recovering from the operation, I made the first sketch. A month later the liver started to undergo chronic rejection. She came to my house and sat for the oil painting on the cover of this book, in which her liver transplants are represented by roses. She then asked me if she could have a fourth liver transplant. I am always amazed that a patient who has gone through such dreadful and painful operative and post-operative procedures would then be prepared to undergo yet another operation.

Fortunately, she recovered from the final operation and has progressed well.

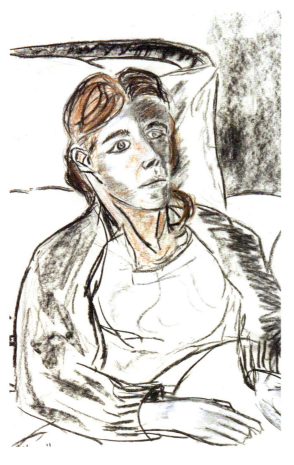

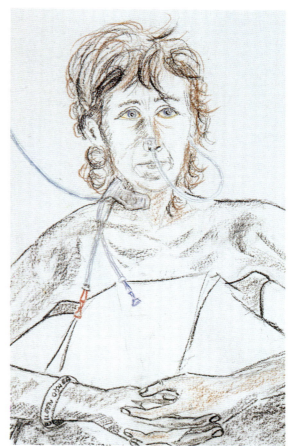

~145~

~146~

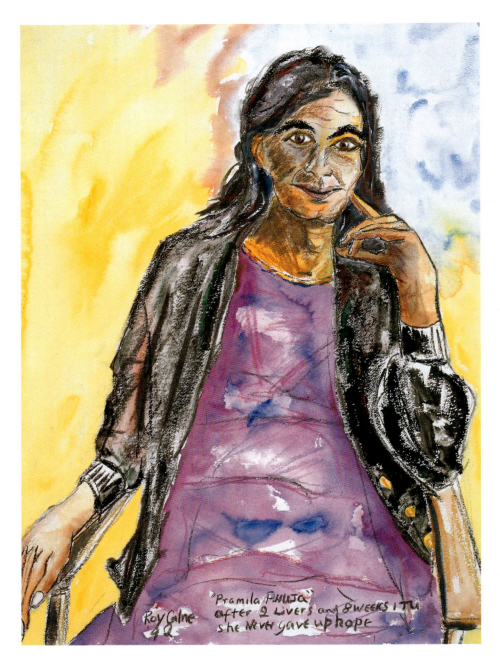

~147~

This lady became extremely ill with pneumonia after her second transplant and required a tracheotomy. Her condition was so poor that she was convinced that she would die. However, the hepatologist, Dr Graeme Alexander, whispered in her ear every day 'don't give up, keep on fighting, you're going to get better'. Later, whilst I was painting her portrait, she told me that these words encouraged her and strengthened her determination to recover.

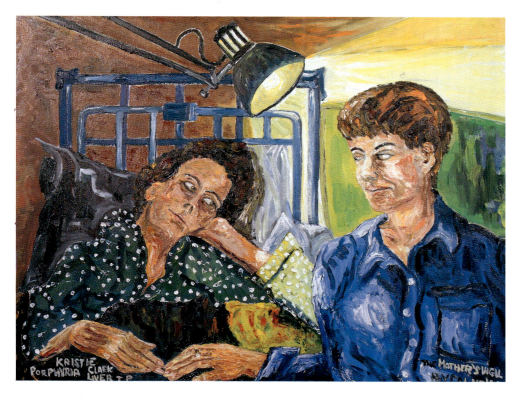

~148~

This girl suffered from porphyria, which is characterised by liver dysfunction and photosensitive lesions on the skin. We therefore transplanted her in an operating room where the main lights were filtered and there were no background lights. The environment was somewhat eerie, justifying the British usage of the words 'operating theatre'. During her recovery, she was nursed in the dark and her mother sat in vigil, night and day, taking care of her.

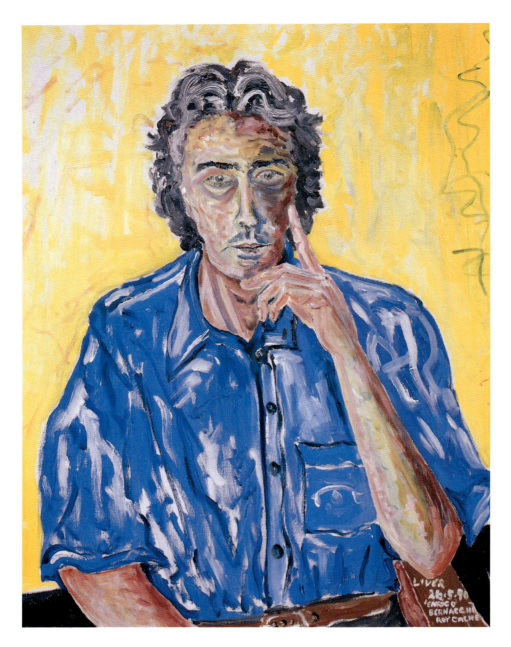

~149~

This man from Italy underwent a liver transplant operation and recovered well. Two years later he came to see me looking extremely sad; I thought something must have gone wrong with his liver, but he explained that his wife (150) needed a liver transplant for a different condition.

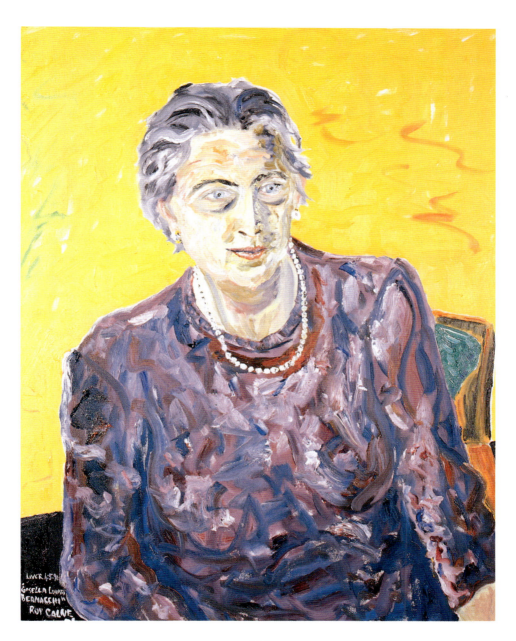

~*150*~

She also received a liver transplant and I painted the husband and wife in the medieval tradition. The paintings were bought, after being exhibited in Singapore, by Mr Seng Tee Lee who subsequently gave them to Wolfson College in Cambridge.

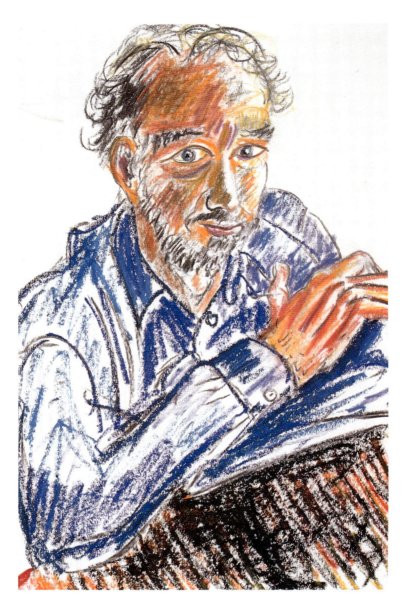

~151~

*John Sherrill Hauser, who received a kidney transplant. He is a distinguished
American artist, whose father was one of the sculptors of the Mount Rushmore
carvings. I had the good fortune to meet him when we had a joint exhibition
in Washington and we painted portraits of each other.*

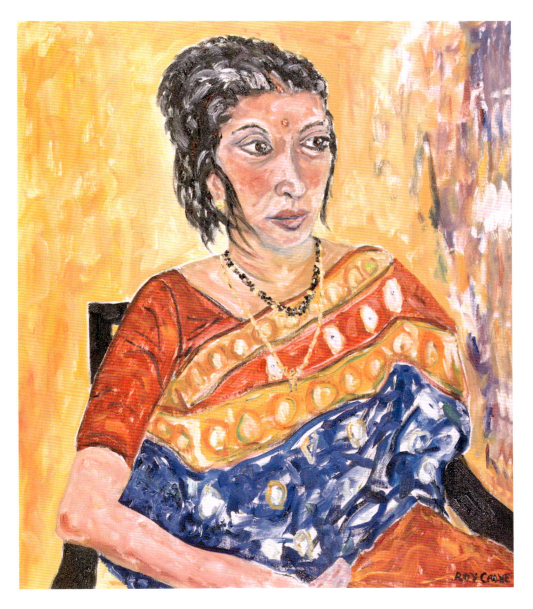

~152~

Dr Sathia Thiru, a distinguished kidney pathologist. She has unrivalled experience of renal transplant histology and over the years has been an essential member of our team. Her knowledge of histology has often meant the difference between success and failure for our patients.

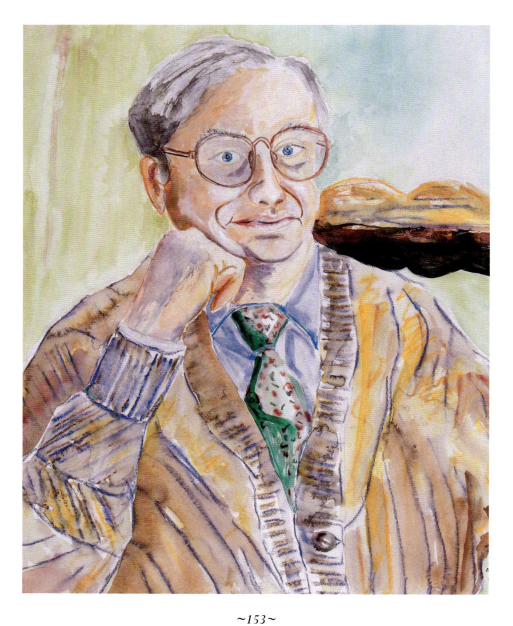

~153~

Dr Suren Sehgal, the discoverer of rapamyzin. He was born in Pakistan, trained in England, and now works in America for Wyeth Ayerst.

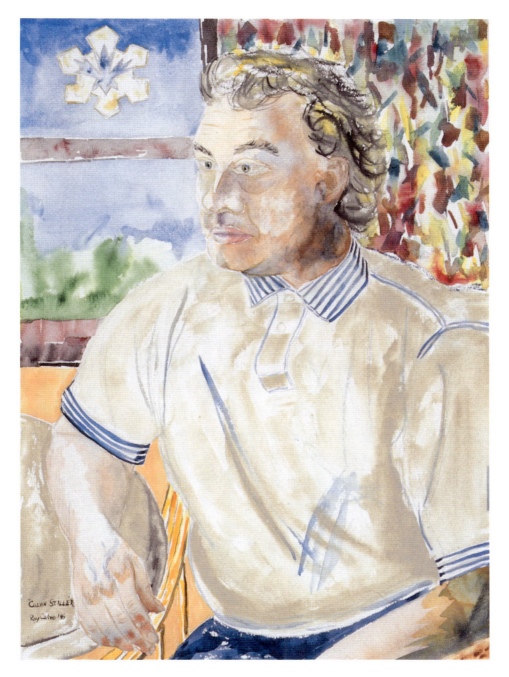

~154~

*Dr Calvin Stiller, nephrologist and Professor at the University of Western
Ontario, Canada. He received the Order of Canada and is responsible for one
of the most respected and excellent transplantation centres in the world.*

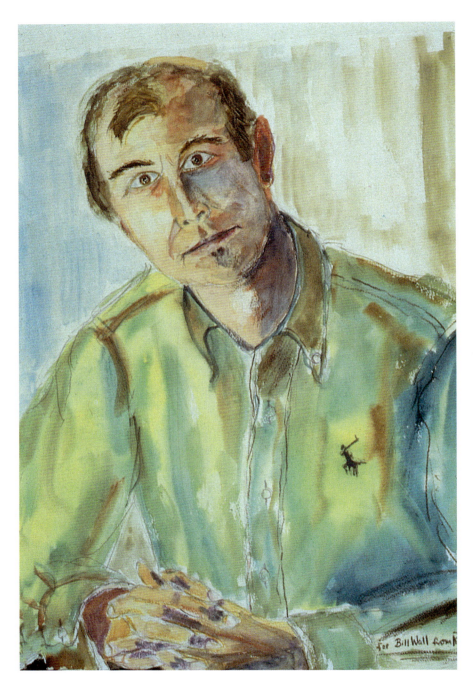

~155~

Dr William Wall, transplant surgeon at the University of Western Ontario, Canada, and a colleague of Dr Stiller. He is an outstanding surgeon and worked in Cambridge with me for two years.

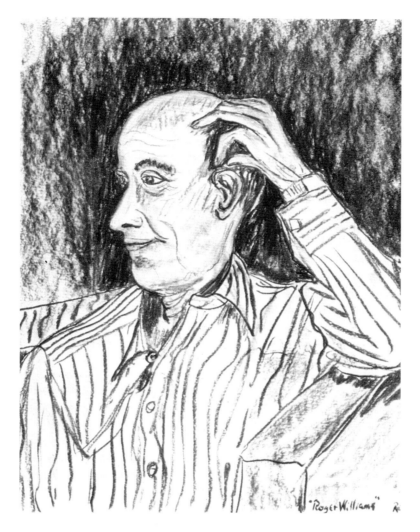

~*156*~

Dr Roger Williams. We worked together at the Royal Free Hospital in 1959
and 1960. Later, I asked him if he would like to join our team in Cambridge.
We worked together for twenty years in both Cambridge and Kings College
Hospital in London. Dr Williams is an internationally renowned hepatologist,
he is also an extremely astute clinician and played a strategic role in the
development of our programme.

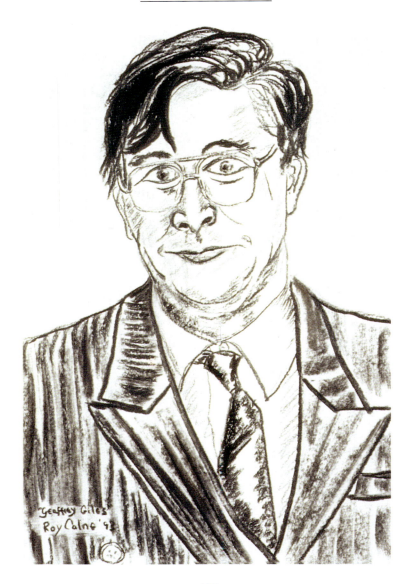

~157~

Professor Geoffrey Giles, Professor of Surgery at the University of Leeds. He trained with Dr Starzl and was an outstanding liver surgeon, who developed an excellent renal transplant programme.

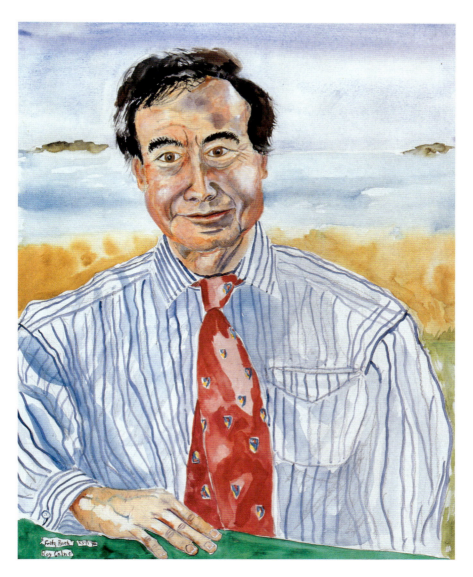

~*158*~

Dr Fritz Bach, one of the pioneers of cellular tissue-typing, particularly human class 2 antigens. He developed a technique for typing patients using a mixed lymphocyte culture reaction, but has now focused his research efforts on xenografting techniques.

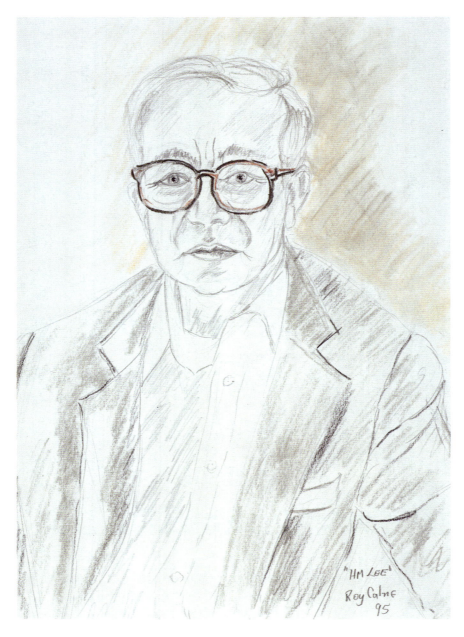

~159~

Dr H M Lee, who worked alongside Dr David Hume at the Medical College of Virginia. He is an outstanding technical surgeon, who has remained in the transplantation field for the past thirty five years.

~160~

Dr Rafael Valdez, Professor of Surgery at the University of Mexico, came to Cambridge as a visiting research fellows and has now established an active transplant unit in Mexico City.

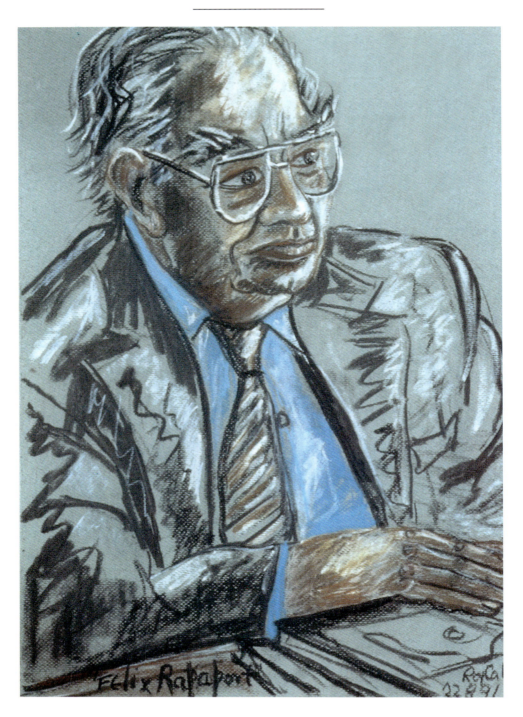

~161~

Dr Felix Rapaport, Professor of Surgery, State University of New York. He is a pioneer of tissue-typing and transplant surgery, and was involved in experimental work with Dr Dausset, concerning the recognition and establishment of the human HLA system.

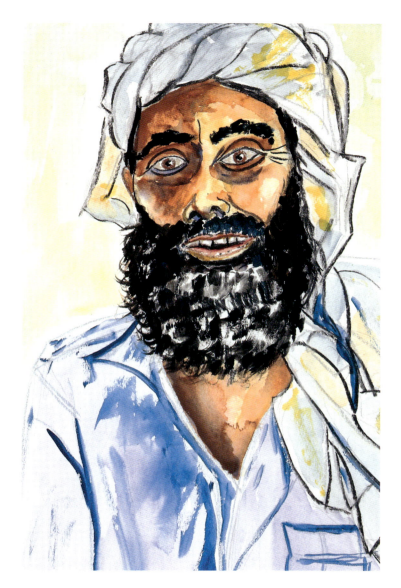

CHAPTER NINE

(162) This gentleman, a patient of Dr Adib Rizvi in Karachi, is the longest surviving recipient of a kidney transplant in Pakistan.

The QUALITY of LIFE
AFTER an ORGAN TRANSPLANT

If a patient receives an organ transplant before irreversible damage has occurred to other parts of the body, the subsequent outcome and the quality of life depend on three main factors:

- controlling rejection so that the organ does not sustain acute or chronic damage

- avoidance of infection, which is important in patients receiving immunosuppressive drugs

- prevention of recurrence of the patient's original disease, whether it is infection, malignancy, auto-immune disease, or the result of alcohol. Congenital defects and diseases due to missing enzymes are usually completely cured by an organ graft.

The overall success rates for transplants of different organs are similar, except those for kidney grafts from living related donors, where there is a higher level of success.

SUCCESS RATES FOR TRANSPLANTS OF
DIFFERENT TYPES OF ORGANS[8]

	GRAFT SURVIVAL (%)		
	1 Year	5 years	10 years
Cadaveric organ grafts	70–80	50–60	40–50
Renal allografts from identically HLA-matched siblings	95	90	85
Renal allografts from 1 haplotype half-matched relative	90	80	70

---

[8]*Update* 19 June 1996 p623 'Transplantation: An update'

Patients requiring organ transplants have often suffered grievously for many years; a successful organ graft may restore them to complete normality. Very often, patients seem to have greater enthusiasm for life than normal and participate in a

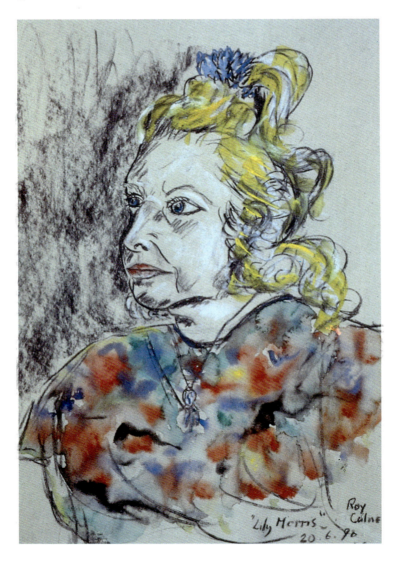

~*163*~

Miss Lilly Morris, a staunch supporter of liver transplantation since her operation in 1988.

(164) This man has received two liver transplants and made a full recovery. He works as a Yeoman Warder at the Tower of London and he was anxious that his medals were correctly depicted when I painted him.

wide range of activities. For example, many transplant patients have participated in the National and International Transplant Olympic Games. This was the brainchild of the transplant surgeon, Maurice Slapak, who felt that the good results of transplantation should be demonstrated by the outstanding rehabilitation of some of the patients.

Of course, not all the patients do so well; some develop unpleasant side effects to the drugs and others are never fully rehabilitated. Complications during the operation may require repeated surgery, or the transplant may fail and need to be replaced. I am always amazed by the courage of the patients,

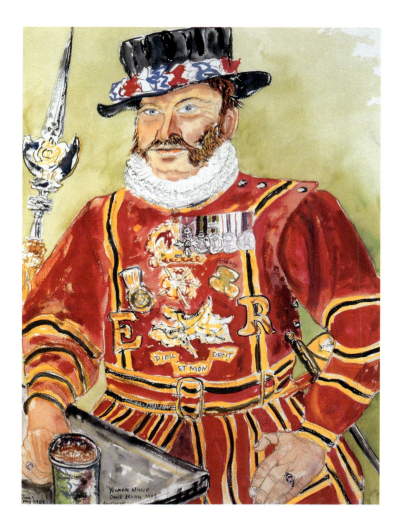

~164~

especially those who undergo several transplant operations. It is the objective of all those working in transplantation to produce graft acceptance without the need for long term immunosuppressive drugs, namely tolerance, or to create an interim phase so that the patient requires only a minimal maintenance dose, without the likelihood of any side effects, "almost tolerance". Some patients with liver grafts have achieved tolerance due to the immunosuppressive effect of the liver.

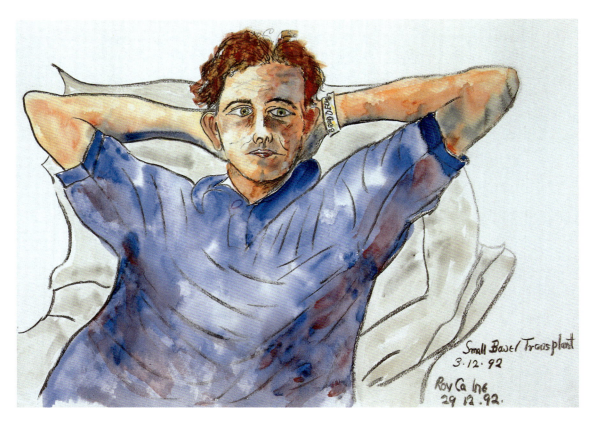

~*165*~

Brad Delve, pictured here, three years after his operation, was the first patient in the UK to undergo an intestinal transplant. When he came out of Intensive Care, the first question he asked me was 'when are you going to paint me?'.

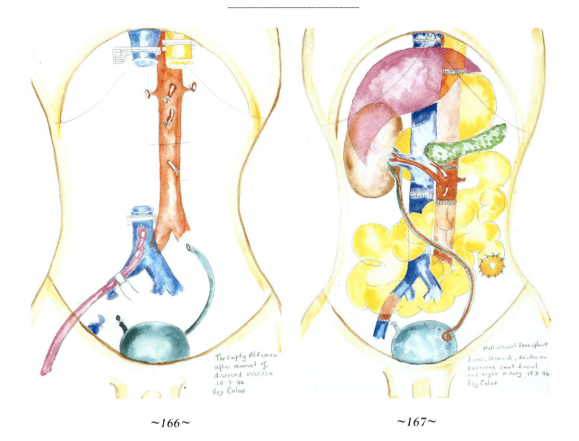

The Empty Abdomen
after removal of
diseased viscera
15.3.94
Roy Calne

Multivisceral Transplant
Liver, stomach, duodenum
pancreas, small bowel
and right kidney 15.3.94
Roy Calne

~166~ ~167~

(166, 167, 168, 169) A patient who had a six-organ transplant for a non-malignant desmoid tumour associated with Gardner's Syndrome. His condition was rapidly deteriorating and he was unable to eat. We explained to him that we did not know whether the operation would be a success. However, a suitable donor was found for all six organs and we offered our patient the chance of a transplant. Three surgeons worked for twelve hours to remove all the diseased organs and the appearance of the abdominal cavity was frightening. When the new en bloc transplant had been finished, he had a new stomach, duodenum, small bowel, liver, pancreas and kidney. The patient's post-operative course was extremely difficult to manage and the ward rounds were cumbersome, involving a gastroenterologist, endocrinologist, hepatologist and nephrologist, as well as a surgeon and, occasionally, a psychiatrist. The patient's stomach took a long time to function, but when it recovered he improved rapidly and is shown in both the recovery phase and six months after the operation. He is now eating properly and is still well two and a half years after the operation, living with his wife and young children. At no time has there been any evidence of rejection in any of the organs, probably due to the effect of the liver and the mass of donor tissue.

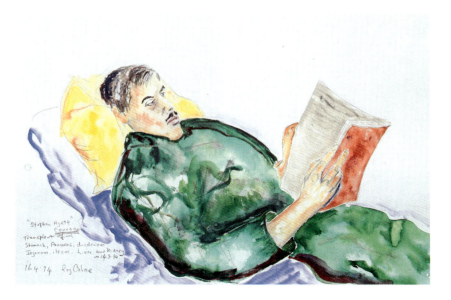

~168~

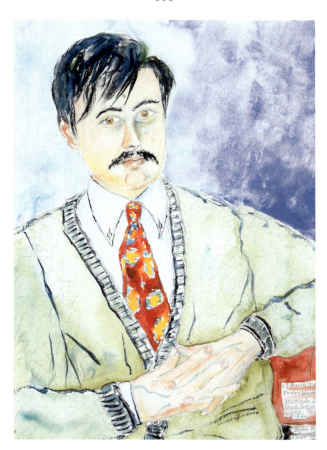

~169~

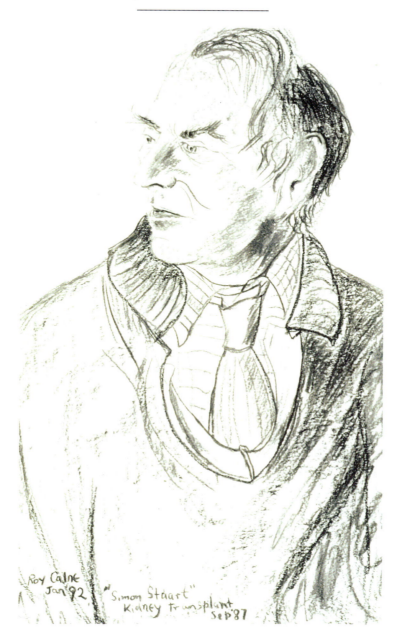

~170~

This patient received a kidney transplant and is pictured here fourteen years
after the operation

There are certainly many difficulties in organ allocation, which may be alleviated by producing animal organs which are suitable for human transplantation. Organ transplantation has been a miracle for many patients, but for others it has been a disappointment. The relatives who have given organs, and the families of patients who have died and whose organs have been used for transplantation, have made extremely generous sacrifices demonstrating human compassion and altruism. For the surgeons involved in organ transplantation, the courage of the patients and their relatives has been the driving force in continuing this work, which has, at times, been harrowing, disappointing and demanding. The saga of transplantation is not over. In the future, patients and their doctors will look back and wonder why we experienced so many setbacks and disappointments.

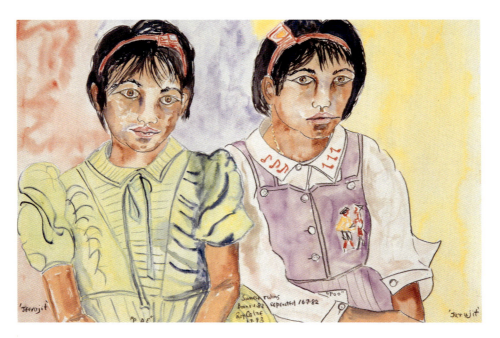

~*171*~

Siamese twins, whom I painted in Bangkok. They were separated at birth and have been brought up in the Red Cross Orphanage of the Chulalongkorn Hospital. They sat absolutely still for twenty minutes while I sketched them and then rushed around with the sketch showing it to all their friends in the orphanage. The painting hangs in the Red Cross Hospital in Bangkok and another version is displayed in Addenbrooke's Hospital, Cambridge.

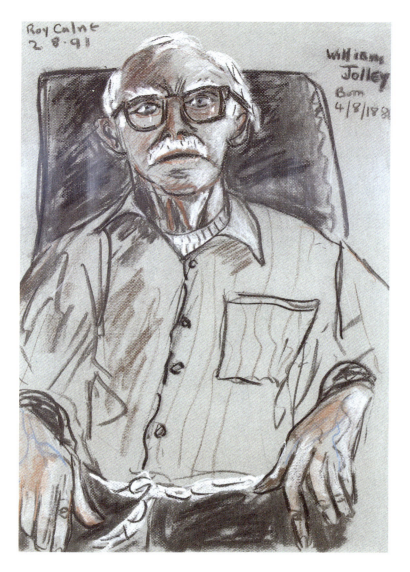

Roy Calne
2 8·91

Williams
Jolley
Born
4/8/18

~172~

Mr William Jolley, pictured here aged 105, was the oldest living soldier in the the UK. He was presented to me with a hernia. I told Mr Jolley that I thought he was too old to have a hernia operation, but he insisted that it bothered him and he would like me to proceed. It was a success and during his recovery period he became so popular with the nurses that they did not want him to go home. Sadly, he has now passed away, but he enjoyed a long and glorious life, to the age of 108.

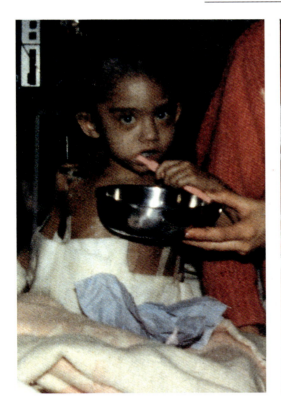

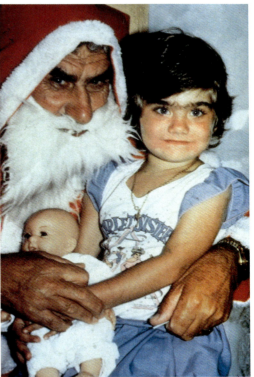

~173~

~174~

(173, 174) Pictures of a child with liver disease before and after undergoing transplantation on Christmas Eve. The following Christmas, the child is hardly recognisable since the change has been so marked.

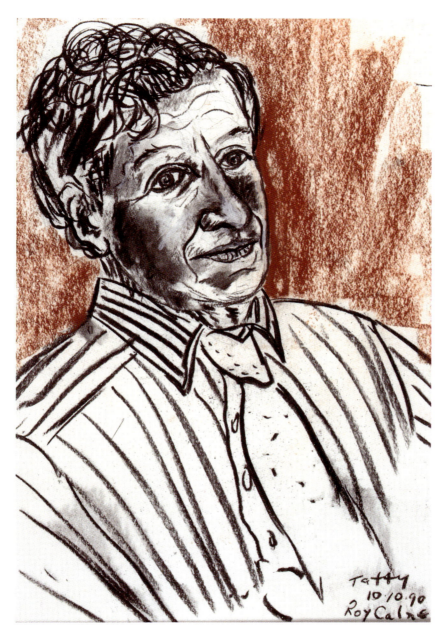

~175~

Mr Maurice (Taffy) Slapak has worked in transplantation research and clinical practice for the past thirty years. It was his idea to establish the Transplant Olympic Games which has been of enormous value in boosting the confidence and self respect of transplant patients. The Transplant Olympics are now an important international event and many countries have their own qualifying athletic meetings.

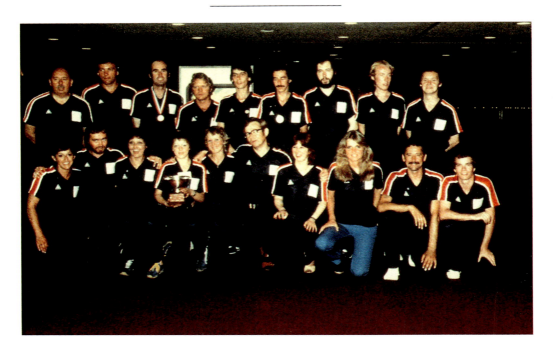

~176~

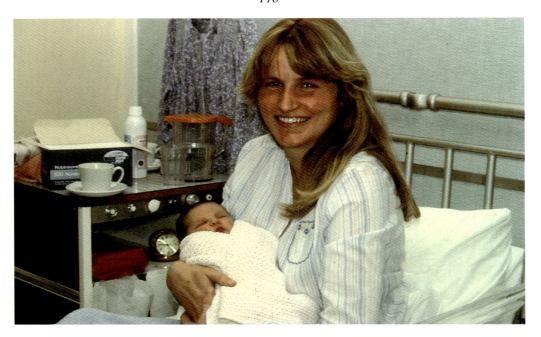

~177~

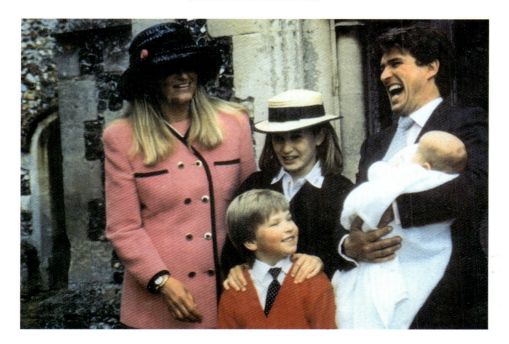

~178~

(176, 177, 178) The British Team who entered the 1980 Transplant Olympics. The girl third from the right in front is shown in the next figure with her first baby and then twelve years later, demonstrating the kind of rehabilitation that is possible after a kidney graft.

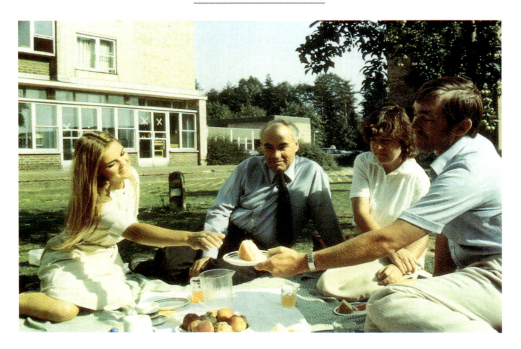

~*179*~

(179, 180, 181) "The forbidden tea-party". After successful pancreas and kidney transplant operations, the patients no longer require insulin injections or regular dialysis and are able to partake of unlimited amounts of orange juice and cake. The girl on the left is shown in the next two figures; the first depicts her with one of her two children born after transplantation and the second shows her with her horse.

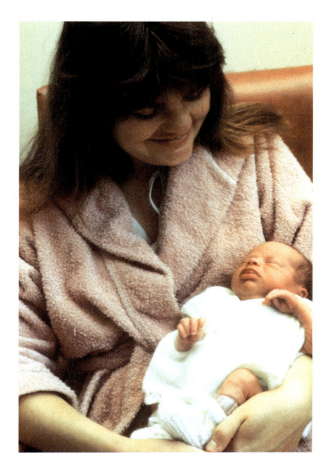

~180~

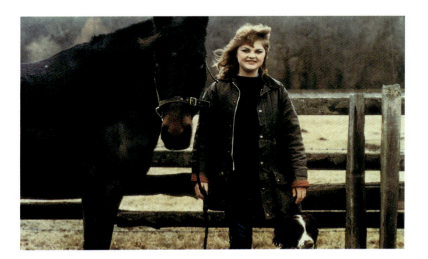

~181~

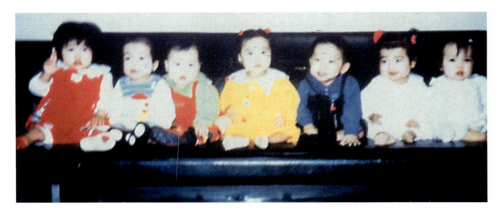

~182~

This photograph was given to me by Dr Yakamara. It shows doll-like Japanese children, who had suffered from congenital biliary atresia and received a liver lobe from one or other parent. This practice has been extensively developed in Japan because of the prevailing law that forbids the use of organs from brain-dead donors. The removal of a lobe of liver is a major sacrifice, but parents seem to be more than willing to volunteer for this.

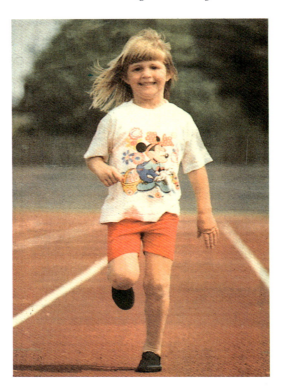

~183~

Girl participating in Transplant Games in Portsmouth, three years after liver transplantation.

ETHICAL *and* MORAL MATTERS

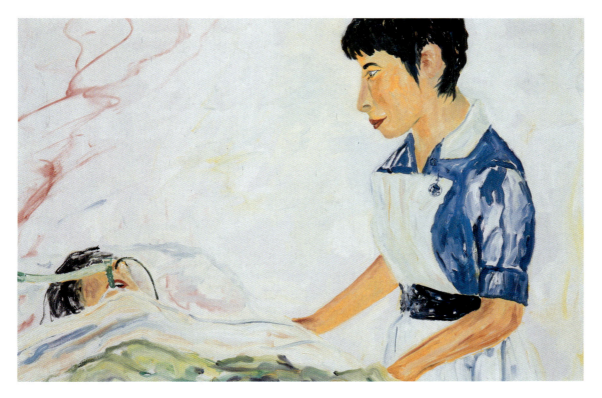

CHAPTER TEN

(184) The Compassion of the Intensive Care Sister. I entered the Intensive Care Ward one evening and saw this Sister looking after an unconscious patient, who was attached to a ventilator. The skill and devotion of the nurse and the one-sided relationship between her and the unconscious patient struck me as a very poignant image. If the patient progresses well he will move out of Intensive Care and if the patient dies the nurse will experience the sadness and bereavement for the family. I know this interpretation is correct because one of my daughters has been an Intensive Care nurse.

TRANSPLANTATION ETHICS

We are faced with many ethical dilemmas concerning organ transplantation, some of which are related to the recipient. We now have access to a number of exceedingly expensive treatments for diseases that had previously been fatal. This is causing concern in every country; even the richest nations cannot afford to provide "high-tech" treatment for every patient who might conceivably benefit, therefore priorities in rationing will be necessary, especially in transplantation surgery. For example, should one transplant the sickest patient, who has the greatest risk of dying during the operation, or should one transplant a patient who is less ill and may fare better?

Surgeons and doctors must discuss each individual case and assess the advantages and disadvantages. One young man was presented to us with a non-malignant tumour strangulating the blood supply of all the organs in his abdomen. His condition was deteriorating rapidly; he was in continuous pain and could not eat normally. After a long discussion with both the patient and his relatives, we decided that although we did not know whether the operation would be successful, we would at least try and help him. When the diseased organs were removed there were no major organs left in the abdominal cavity. After his six-organ transplant his condition was very unstable and he was difficult to look after, but he recovered from this procedure without any evidence of rejection of the grafted organs, probably due to the protective effect of the liver. He is now well, two and a half years after transplantation (figures 166–169).

There are also ethical worries concerning the nature of a patient's disease. We were contemplating operating on a patient with alcoholic liver disease. Although he had given up drinking our nurses felt that this was an unethical operation. Discussion may not have resolved the ethical issue, but at least we showed that it was not a simple matter. A doctor, by reason of traditional medical ethics, is obliged to do the best possible for every patient, regardless of whether he approves of their lifestyle. We have no qualms in treating a road accident victim caused by reckless driving. We may feel less happy about treating a road traffic accident victim if he had stolen the car under the influence of drugs and killed children waiting at a bus stop. I do not pretend to have a clear ethical opinion on this matter, except to say that the doctor still should do his best for the patient who comes to him for treatment.

Consideration of the donor is of paramount importance in any transplant operation. If the donor is alive, for instance a parent giving a kidney to a child, there are ethical concerns and it is important that both the patient and the donor realise that the operation is not without risk. There is a very small chance of death of the donor and a very much higher chance of morbidity. Even with a good tissue match and modern drugs, rejection can still occur. Contact between the recipient and donor's relatives in cadaver donation is not generally encouraged, but sometimes it has resulted in a precious friendship between the two families.

The care of patients undergoing transplantation is complicated and expensive, but the devotion and compassion of the Intensive Care nurses is quite exceptional. They have enormous skill, knowledge and their patients are unconscious for most of the time they are looking after them. Following recovery the patient is rapidly transferred to a less specialised ward and if the patient dies this is an added sadness after so much professional and emotional effort.

I am much more concerned about live organ donation between individuals who are not blood relatives. Terasaki has shown that transplants between husband and wife are very successful. This surprising finding has caused a sudden major increase in spouse to spouse kidney grafting in the United States. However, this has raised an interesting medico-legal question; since the overall incidence of divorce is approximately 30%, some people are concerned as to how a kidney donation would fare in a divorce settlement. In one of his recent talks, Dr Terasaki showed a slide of a hypothetical statement from a wife to the husband "yes you can have my kidney in return for a fast divorce, the house, your Ferrari and an annual income of $200,000". This extreme fictional case would be the same as paying for a kidney from an unrelated donor, a procedure that is considered unethical by the International Transplantation Society.

It is not surprising that as the results of transplantation get better, the demand increases and this is the main stimulus for xenograft research. Surgeons hope that the manipulation of animal species, perhaps by transgenic procedures, will result in donor organs that are acceptable to Man.

There is no doubt that transplant surgery is expensive and the costs incurred are often challenged by healthcare economists. For the patients who do well, it is a marvellous form of treatment and some of them return to a completely normal life. Others have been hospitalised so long, or experienced complications that render them physically and/or mentally incapable of rehabilitation. If we only look at transplant surgery and, indeed, all "high-tech" medicine and surgery from the point of view of expenditure, the returns would seem to be poor: however, the public perception of advances is a very important matter in a democratic country. Adequate funding will never be obtained and there will always be cries for more money. Therefore, some form of prioritisation will inevitably be necessary.

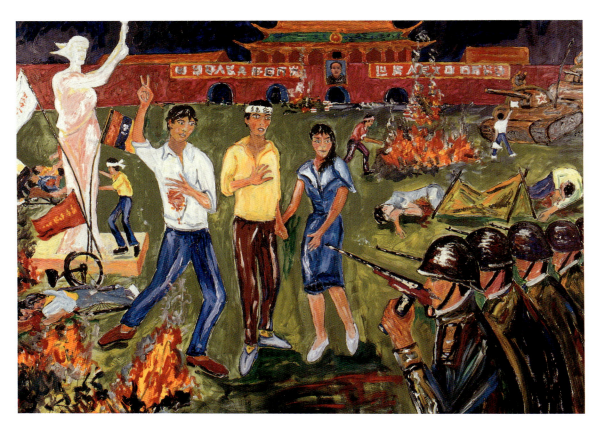

~185~

An impression of the massacre of students in Tiananmen Square. Goya in his famous 3rd of May painting depicted a martyr being callously shot by impersonal soldiers. Manet also used this theme in his painting of the execution of Emperor Maximillian in Mexico. In the background is a statue of liberty that the students made. The torch is held by two hands as the students explained that liberty is so difficult to come by in China that two hands were needed to hold the torch. Sadly the flame of hope went out the night the tanks rumbled on top of the defenceless students.

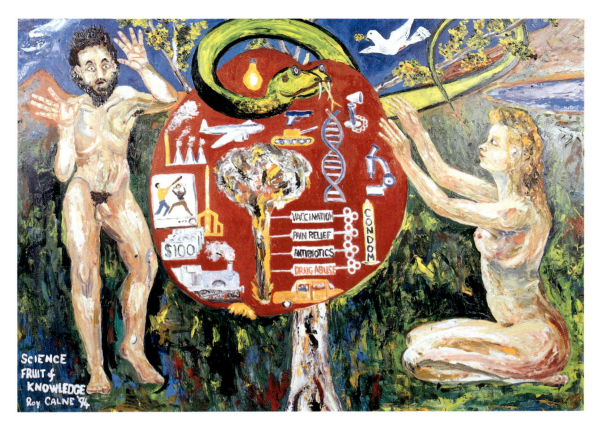

~186~

This painting of "Science" was commissioned by the Science Museum in London. It was the frontispiece of my book *Too Many People* (published by Calder Publications Ltd.). It shows Eve receiving the fruit of the Tree of Knowledge from the serpent with DNA coming from his fangs and good and bad applications of Science, which itself is morally neutral. Indicated are immunisation, pain relief, antibiotics, the evil of drug abuse, violence in the media, pollution of the air, corruption, arms. The applications of Science that are neither good nor bad are included; electricity, flying, the internal combustion engine, the steam engine, microscope and the telephone and the need for effective birth control – a condom. In the centre is the nuclear bomb. Adam seems worried at the prospect of accepting this gift. My mother-in-law saw the painting and insisted that the painting was so sad there must be a dove bringing hope, hence my mother-in-law's dove.

In the book *Too Many People*, I expounded my theory of control of population as a means to conserving the world's resources. With the progress of science has come great advances in biology and medicine and potentially destructive advances in scientific weapons. The understanding of DNA is the key to our past and future, and renders us capable of producing the best and the worst in Man.

HYPOTHESIS

The Creator's Testament to Modern Man

I have given you DNA programmed by evolution through millions of years. It has form, function and instincts derived from your anthropoid ancestors. You have evolved the gift of language and intelligence to possess the ability to reason, to enquire, to have abstract thoughts from which you may experience rich emotions. These blessings bestowed on you are to be used to live in peace with fellow-men, animals, plants and the elements of the earth.

From your ancestors you have inherited the urge to reproduce to preserve your precious DNA. Many of the secrets of nature are now revealed to you by your probing curiosity and rational analysis. This knowledge can be used for good or evil.

The legend of the serpent who gave Eve the fruit of knowledge is a terrible warning; beware not to succumb to the temptations of greed, envy, fanatic hatred and lust for power to dominate others. If you continue to multiply without constraint or consideration of the rest of the world you will swiftly exhaust irreplaceable resources, animal, vegetable and mineral, which will surely lead to the destruction of your DNA and the desolation of the planet.

You will have many hard decisions to make but I have given you the ability to choose. In the spirit of love and compassion towards your fellow men and all living creatures, animals, and plants, use your scientific knowledge to choose and act wisely to devise ways of sharing without exploitation, to live and let live.

I hope you become *Homo SAPIENS,* the alternative is *Homo EXTINCTUS.*

PERMISSIONS LIST

Figures 2, 3, 4, 5 and 6
Self-Portrait with Helen (1987), Bonjour Professor Calne, Addenbrooke's Hospital (1988), Convalescence, all by John Bellany. Kind permission of the artist, from the Collection of the National Galleries of Scotland, Edinburgh.

Figure 10
The Illustrated History of Surgery, by Knut Haeger, Harold Starke Publishers Limited, Suffolk, England.

Figure 11
Grottes Chauvet, France
Science, Vol 267, 3 February 1995.

Figure 12
Horse Running, Lascaux Caves, France
Robert Harding Picture Library, London

Figure 16
Circumcision in ancient Egypt
Wellcome Institute Library, London

Figure 17
Musei Civici, Piacenza, Italy

Figure 34
Peale: Venus Rising from the Sea – A Deception (After the Bath), ca. 1822
The Nelson-Atkins Museum of Art, Kansas City, Missouri, USA (Purchase: Nelson Trust)

Figures 48 and 49
From a collection of anatomical drawings by Leonardo da Vinci
The Royal Collection, Her Majesty The Queen

Figure 50
Vesalius: Lateral view of a skeleton, contemplating a skull.
Wellcome Institute Library, London

Figure 51
Leonardo da Vinci: Head of a Woman
The Royal Collection, Her Majesty The Queen

Figure 52
Rembrandt van Rijn: The Anatomy Lesson of Dr. Nicolas Tulp
"Mauritshuis", The Hague, The Netherlands

Figure 53
Francisco Goya: Portrait of Goya Sick (1820)
Seligman Collection, Paris

Figure 54
Gabriel Metsu: The Sick Child (1660)
Rijksmuseum
Amsterdam, The Netherlands

Figure 55
Edward Munch: The Sick Child
Tate Gallery, London

Figure 56
Albrecht Dürer: Self-Portrait meant for the Doctor
Kunsthalle Bremen
Bremen, Germany

Figure 57
Rembrandt van Rijn: Bethsébée au bain (1654)
Musée du Louvre, Paris

Figure 58
Drawing by William Skelton from *The Cause and Effects of the Variolae Vaccine*, by Edward Jenner, London 1798.

Figure 59
Injection Specimen of the Spinal Cord
from *An Atlas of Vascular Anatomy of the Skeleton and Spinal Cord*, by Henry Vernon Crock, Martin Dunitz, London, 1996. By kind permission of the author.

Figure 62
Vincent van Gogh: Le docteur Paul Gachet (1890)
Musée d'Orsay, Paris

Figure 63
Vincent van Gogh: Self-Portrait with one ear cut off
Courtauld Institute Galleries, London

Figure 64
Doctor Gachet: Charcoal Portrait of Vincent van Gogh on his death bed
Collection of Paul Gachet

Figure 65
Henry Tonks: Underground Casualty Clearing Station, Cat No 1653.
Collection: Imperial War Museum, London. Copyright: The Artists Estate.

Figure 66
Henry Tonks: Injured Face before plastic surgery
From a collection of drawings by Henry Tonks
The Royal College of Surgeons of England

Figures 67 and 68
from Charles Bell: Essays on the Anatomy of Expression in Painting
London 1806

Figure 69
Charles Bell: Soldier Dying from Tetanus
The Royal College of Surgeons of Edinburgh, Scotland

Figure 71
Frida Kahlo: The Broken Column (1944)
Collection of Dolores Olmedo, Mexico City

Figure 72
Frida Kahlo: Tree of Hope (1946)
Collection of Daniel Filipacchi, Paris

Figure 73
Frida Kahlo: Portrait of Dr. Leo Eleosser (1931)
University of California, San Francisco School of Medicine, San Francisco, California, USA

Figures 75 and 76
"First Patient Interview" and "Informal Meeting in Medical School Cafeteria"
May Lesser: An Artist in the University Medical Center
Tulane University Press, 1989, New Orleans, Louisiana.
Courtesy of the artist.

Figure 77
Joseph Wilder: Contemplation Before Surgery (1987)
As published in Surgical Reflections, Quality Medical Publishing, St. Louis, Missouri, USA

Figure 78
Max Beckmann: Drawing of Ferdinand Sauerbruch
Collection of Peter Sauerbruch, Bonn Germany

Figure 80
Alice Neal: Last Sickness
Journal of the American Medical Association, May 6, 1992, V 267, No 17.

Figure 81
Thomas Eakins: The Gross Clinic (1875)
Thomas Jefferson University, Philadelphia, Pennsylvania, USA

Figure 82
Thomas Eakins: The Agnew Clinic (1889)
University of Pennsylvania, School of Medicine, Philadelphia, Pennsylvania, USA

Figures 83 and 84
Fra Angelica: The Miracle of Saints Cosmos and Damian
Museo di San Marco, Firenze, Italy

Figure 85
Mantegna: Diptych of Saints Cosmos and Damian
Society of Antiquaries of London, London

Figure 130
Ralph Steadman: "Napoleon" illustration from George Orwell's Animal Farm
Reed Books, London. By kind permission of the artist.

Figures 173, 174, 177–182
Photographs by kind permission of the individuals.

Figure 176
Courtesy of Maurice Slapak.

Figure 186
Roy Calne: Science: The Fruit of the Tree of Knowledge
The Science Museum, London

Text (Hypothesis)
The author and publishers thank Professor Sir Roy Calne and the Calder Educational Trust, London, for permission to Reprint "Hypothesis" from Too Many People by Roy Calne, published by Calder Publications Ltd., London, and Riverrun Press Inc., New York. Copyright © Roy Calne 1994.

Back cover Figure
John Hauser: Drawing of Roy Calne
Courtesy of the artist.

All proceeds of sales of paintings by Sir Roy Calne benefit the
Children's Liver Transplant Research Fund.